Tools for
Community Planning
Group Members

HIV Prevention Community Planning: *An Orientation Guide*

January 2005

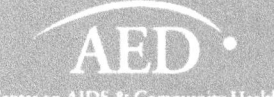

Center on AIDS & Community Health

Developed by the AED Center on AIDS & Community Health with funding provided by the Centers for Disease Control and Prevention under contract #200-97-0605 task 084.

Tools for
Community Planning
Group Members

HIV Prevention
Community Planning:
An Orientation Guide

January 2005

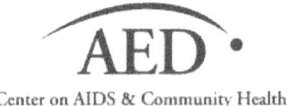

Center on AIDS & Community Health

*Developed by the AED Center on AIDS & Community Health with
funding provided by the Centers for Disease Control and
Prevention under contract #200-97-0605 task 084.*

HIV Prevention

Table of Contents

Acknowledgments

We would like to acknowledge Janet Cleveland, Robert Kohmescher, Corinne Matthews, and Sam Taveras at the Centers for Disease Control and Prevention (CDC), Division of HIV/AIDS Prevention, for their support during the development phase of this guide.

The main authors were Denise Raybon and Gary B. MacDonald of the Academy for Educational Development (AED). Additional AED contributors included Margaret Anderson, Nickie Bazell, Frank Beadle de Palomo, Sharon Novey, James Testaverde, Scott Thompson, and Joy Workman.

Anne Rodgers served as senior editor. Jean Kohanek and Jose Noda of AED designed the document. Additional reviewers included: Catherine Hulburt, Kathy Donner, Liatris Studer, Lynne Greabell, Aurturo Ponce, and Ed Tepporn.

Miguel Santos Gonzalez served as Spanish Translator.

AED's Center on AIDS & Community Health prepared this document under contract to the Centers for Disease Control and Prevention (contract #200-97-0605, task #084) to provide technical assistance and support for HIV prevention community planning.

Introduction

HIV Prevention Community Planning: An Orientation Guide is a companion to the Centers for Disease Control & Prevention (CDC's) 2004-2008 *Guidance for HIV Prevention Community Planning* (called "the *Guidance*" from now on). This guide brings information together in simple language that individual users need to know about HIV Prevention Community Planning by:

- Providing a brief background on the history and guiding principles of HIV Prevention Community Planning and how it is evolving in response to CDC's Advancing HIV Prevention Initiative (AHP);

- Describing the roles and responsibilities of the key community planning players — Community Planning Group (CPG) members, health departments, and the CDC;

- Explaining the community planning process — the products you and your CPG partners need to complete in order to prepare a Comprehensive HIV Prevention Plan;

- Discussing the processes used by many CPGs to manage their work effectively; and

- Describing monitoring and evaluation activities that are necessary to ensure that the goals and objectives of community planning are met, including those of the CPG, health department, and CDC.

How Does This Orientation Guide Differ From the *Guidance*?

The *Guidance* is sometimes called the "blueprint" of community planning. It contains the information you need to know about the community planning process. The *Guidance* was developed by CDC in collaboration with CPGs, health departments, and other national partners. This collaboration reflects one of the guiding principles of community planning: working together.

CDC issued the first version of this blueprint for HIV Prevention Community Planning in December 1993 and has updated it twice since then. The latest version is the 2004-2008 *Guidance for HIV Prevention Community Planning*. The *Guidance* is designed to give flexible direction to state, local, and territorial health departments on how to design and implement a participatory community planning process. It includes sections on:

- The Importance of HIV Prevention Community Planning

- Community Planning Goals and Objectives

- The Planning Process

- The Comprehensive HIV Prevention Plan and Key Products

- Monitoring and Evaluation

- Roles and Responsibilities

- Accountability

Getting the Most out of CDC's *Guidance*

The 2004-2008 *Guidance for HIV Prevention Community Planning* is essential to your participation in the planning process. **Before using this orientation guide, be sure to read the *Guidance* cover to cover:**

- Reading the *Guidance* will empower you to be an effective member of your CPG. The *Guidance* provides you with all the information you need to understand your role in the CPG and the planning process.

- Mark sections that you find useful, refer to your specific role, or are passages you think you'll want to refer to later. Go back to these sections often.

- Highlight any information you don't understand and ask questions about these sections. Ask your CPG co-chairs for explanations or encourage your CPG to allow time for questions at each meeting. If your CPG has not held a new member orientation yet, ask when the next one will be conducted.

HIV Prevention Community Planning: An Orientation Guide covers the same topics as the *Guidance* but in simpler language. We hope it will be a useful overview to help you learn more about the community planning process, products, and expected outcomes. However, this document is not intended to replace the *Guidance*. If you have questions about any aspect of HIV Prevention Community Planning, always consult the *Guidance* as the authority.

When you've finished reading this document, see how much you've learned and what questions you still have. **Fill out the "Community Planning Orientation Self-Assessment Checklist" in Appendix A.**

How is this Document Organized?

This guide is organized to help you quickly and easily find the information you need.

The guide also contains several useful **Appendices**:

- Appendix A: Community Planning Orientation Self-Assessment Checklist

- Appendix B: Summary of the Changes in the 2004-2008 *Guidance for HIV Prevention Community Planning*

- Appendix C: Putting the "P" in PIR: Tips for Orienting Your CPG

- Appendix D: Sample Letters of Concurrence, Concurrence with Reservations, and Non-Concurrence

- Appendix E: Critical Attributes of HIV Prevention Community Planning

- Appendix F: Community Planning Monitoring and Evaluation Forms

- Appendix G: Additional Resources for Community Planning Groups

Also, check out **www.hivaidsta.org** for publications, tools, links, peer samples, and a listserv.

INTRODUCTION

HIV Prevention Community Planning: An Orientation Guide

1

What Is HIV Prevention Community Planning and How Has It Changed?

HIV Prevention Community Planning is a process in which people from different walks of life and different interests, responsibilities, and involvement in HIV prevention come together as a group to plan how to prevent HIV infection where they live.

In most places, this planning group is called a Community Planning Group (CPG). CPGs are a partnership between state, local, or territorial health departments and community members who are infected with and affected by HIV. One of the roles of the health department is to fund HIV prevention programs in their state, city, or territory. Community members can be community advocates, agency directors, educators, outreach workers, relatives of people living with HIV — usually a very diverse group. Most important, CPG members should always include people living with HIV and those at high risk of infection.

A diverse membership that represents the jurisdiction's prevention populations is important because it helps CPGs design local prevention plans that focus on the real-life, specific needs of people at risk of, or living with, HIV. CPGs use a variety of methods to achieve such a membership. New members may be recruited through service agencies or through a Ryan White Planning Council. Other recruitment methods may include word-of-mouth; seeking volunteers at health fairs and community forums; and radio, TV, and newspaper ads.

Why Was HIV Prevention Community Planning Necessary?

In the days before HIV Prevention Community Planning, communities were *doing* HIV prevention activities but they were not often involved in *planning* comprehensive state and local prevention activities. Decisions about HIV prevention were usually made at the national level — either required by Congress or directed by the U.S. Centers for Disease Control and Prevention (CDC) through funding agreements with state, local, or territorial health departments. CDC is the chief government agency responsible for HIV prevention activities in the United States.

HIV Prevention Community Planning was instituted based on the belief that **local** decision making is the best way to respond to local HIV prevention needs and priorities.

What Do Community Planning Groups Do?

The primary task of the CPG is to work with territorial, state, or local health departments to develop a Comprehensive HIV Prevention Plan that is based on scientific evidence and community needs. Through its descriptions of priority populations and ongoing services and recommendations about prevention interventions, the Plan is intended to guide a jurisdiction's response to the HIV epidemic. The Comprehensive HIV Prevention Plan should describe the jurisdiction's entire HIV prevention program. This is what "comprehensive" means: all prevention activities and interventions, regardless of funding source. This means that CPGs should recommend activities and interventions that will be funded by federal funds as well as those funded by other sources, including the state or locality or non-governmental funders, such as foundations. As a result, CPGs should know and understand the full range of prevention resources available in the jurisdiction and how these resources are allocated.

To develop a Comprehensive Prevention Plan, the CPG must complete a process that includes:

- Assessing the impact of the epidemic in their localities (the Epidemiologic Profile);

- Describing the prevention needs of populations living with or at risk of HIV infection,

---

What do we mean by "Jurisdiction?"

A jurisdiction is the CPG's geographic or service area. CDC funds 65 jurisdictions, which include:

- All 50 states

- The District of Columbia

- Six directly-funded cities (Chicago, Houston, Los Angeles, New York, Philadelphia, San Francisco)

- Puerto Rico, the U.S. Virgin Islands, and six U.S. affiliated Pacific Island jurisdictions (American Samoa, Commonwealth of the Northern Mariana Islands, Federated States of Micronesia, Guam, Republic of Palau, and Republic of the Marshall Islands)

the prevention activities and interventions being carried out to address these needs and gaps in existing services (the Community Services Assessment);

- Prioritizing a set of target populations (identified through the Epidemiologic Profile and Community Services Assessment) who require prevention efforts because of their high rates of HIV infection and strong evidence of risky behaviors; and

- Defining a set of prevention activities and interventions (based on intervention effectiveness and cultural/ethnic appropriateness) that are necessary to reduce HIV transmission in target populations.

The health department uses this Comprehensive HIV Prevention Plan as the basis for its annual application to CDC for federal HIV prevention funding. In addition, many states use the Plan to allocate state resources and as a tool to guide other funders.

What is PIR?

A fundamental component of the HIV prevention community planning process is parity, inclusion, and representation (often referred to as PIR). All three concepts are intended to ensure that CPGs include a diverse group of members who truly understand and represent those most affected by the epidemic. PIR is also intended to ensure that every member is able to participate and have a voice in what happens.

Parity means that all members can participate and carry out planning tasks. To achieve parity, all members must get an orientation to community planning (see Appendix C: Tips for Orienting Your CPG), have opportunities to learn and build community planning skills, and have a voice in making decisions.

Inclusion is defined as meaningful involvement of members in the process with an active voice in decision-making. An inclusive process assures that the views, perspectives, and needs of all affected communities are included.

Representation is the act of serving as an official member reflecting the perspective of a specific community. A representative should truly reflect the perspective of that community's values, beliefs, and behaviors. It is also important, however, that representatives are able to participate objectively in the overall prioritization process.

What Are the Guiding Principles, Goals, and Objectives of Community Planning?

It is important that the community planning process is carried out in a way that ensures participation reflecting the jurisdiction's epidemic. It also needs to do its work effectively. To make sure this happens, CDC expects all CPGs to abide by a specific set of guiding principles (see the *Guidance*, Section IID, for full explanations of each principle) and to address a specific set of planning goals, objectives, and attributes. Figure 1 presents an overview of community planning principles, the goals, and their corresponding objectives.

FIGURE 1.

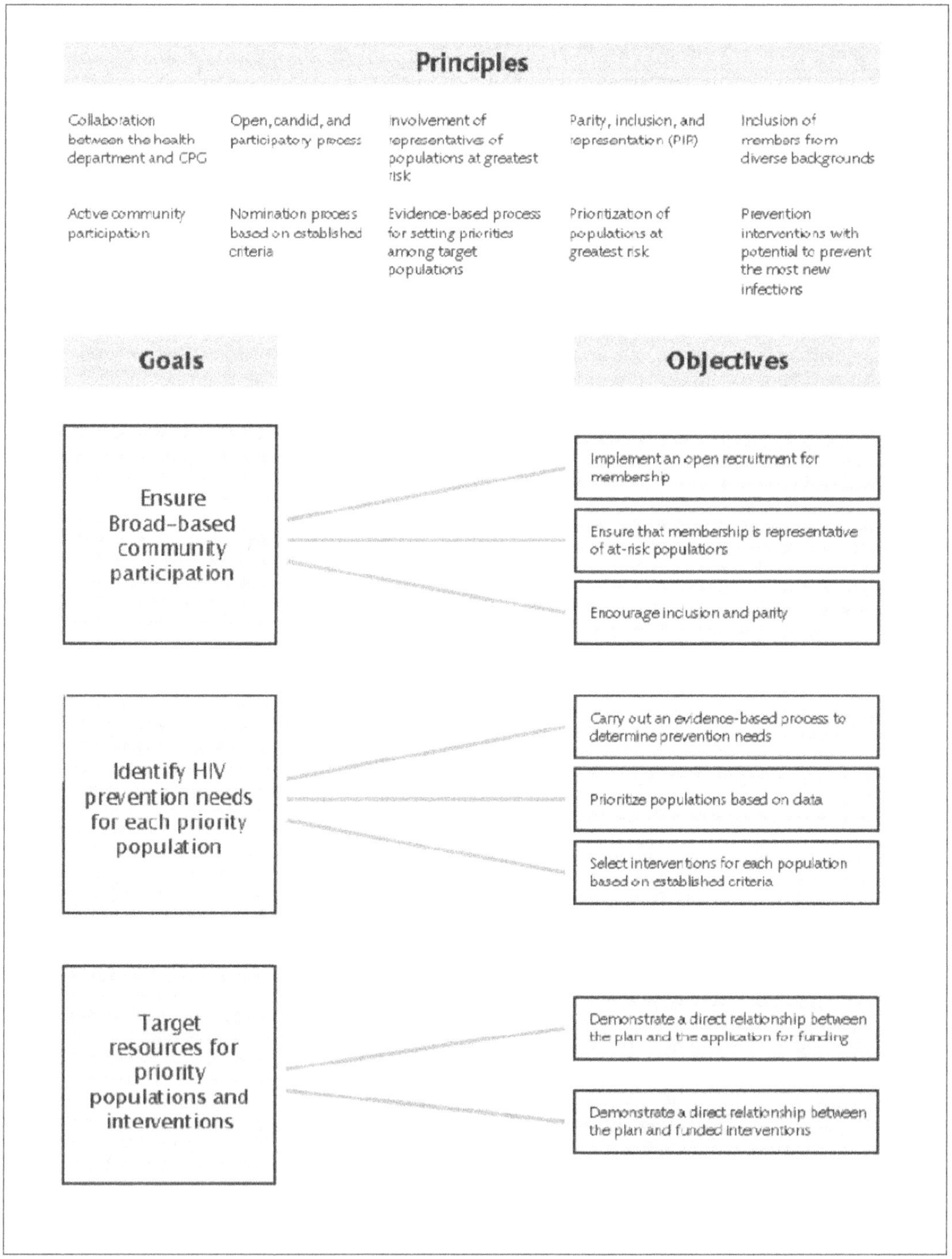

Principles

Collaboration between the health department and CPG

Open, candid, and participatory process

Involvement of representatives of populations at greatest risk

Parity, inclusion, and representation (PIR)

Inclusion of members from diverse backgrounds

Active community participation

Nomination process based on established criteria

Evidence-based process for setting priorities among target populations

Prioritization of populations at greatest risk

Prevention interventions with potential to prevent the most new infections

Goals

Objectives

Ensure Broad-based community participation

Implement an open recruitment for membership

Ensure that membership is representative of at-risk populations

Encourage inclusion and parity

Identify HIV prevention needs for each priority population

Carry out an evidence-based process to determine prevention needs

Prioritize populations based on data

Select interventions for each population based on established criteria

Target resources for priority populations and interventions

Demonstrate a direct relationship between the plan and the application for funding

Demonstrate a direct relationship between the plan and funded interventions

How Has Community Planning Changed Over Time?

With the development of the 2004-2008 *Guidance*, the community planning process has undergone several changes. The table in Appendix B describes these changes in detail, and the following paragraphs provide a summary.

A new focus on the overall planning process and key products, not planning "steps."
Community planning previously emphasized nine steps in the planning process. This suggested that the planning process was linear — one step following another. However, actual experience showed that many parts of the planning process occur at the same time. Community planning now emphasizes the overall process and the products that result from that process.

The new Community Services Assessment. Under the previous *Guidance*, CPGs were responsible for developing three products: a local needs assessment, a resource inventory, and an analysis of gaps in services. Under the current *Guidance*, these activities have been combined and are now referred to as a Community Services Assessment (CSA). Responsibility for conducting the CSA is now primarily the role of the health department with input and review from CPGs. However, it is important to ensure that the CPG is still actively involved in the assessment process. The CPG might help determine the scope, guide the questions to be asked and in some cases, participate in implementation of the assessment.

Changes to priority setting. Under the previous *Guidance*, the Comprehensive HIV Prevention Plan had to rank priority target populations as well as priority HIV prevention activities and interventions. Under the current *Guidance*, the Plan must still identify and prioritize specific populations, but CPGs are no longer required to prioritize interventions. CPGs are now required to identify a set of interventions for each population.

A greater emphasis on monitoring and evaluation. Under the current *Guidance*, monitoring and evaluating the planning process are much more structured and well-defined activities than before. CPGs and health departments are expected to use concrete indicators and tools to monitor the process and report on its effectiveness.

Community Planning and CDC's Advancing HIV Prevention Initiative

In recent years, several aspects of the HIV/AIDS epidemic have come together to create the impetus for CDC's Advancing HIV Prevention (AHP) Initiative. The first is that declines in HIV/AIDS illness and death rates have ended, and data suggest that the annual number of new HIV infections in some populations may be increasing. Another aspect is the fact that up to one-quarter of the 850,000 to 950,000 people infected with HIV do not know that they are infected. The third aspect is the recent approval of a new rapid HIV test.

AHP addresses these developments by reducing barriers to early diagnosis of HIV infection and helping people get into quality medical care, treatment, and prevention services. CPG members need to be familiar with the AHP initiative because it will have a direct impact on community planning. Through AHP, CDC is refocusing some HIV prevention activities so as to put more emphasis on:

- HIV counseling, testing, and referral;

- Notification of partners of people infected with HIV;

- Prevention services for people living with HIV; and

- Routine, universal HIV screening as a part of prenatal care.

CDC has four strategies for achieving AHP objectives:

Strategy 1: Make HIV testing a routine part of medical care.

Strategy 2: Develop and encourage models for diagnosing HIV infections outside medical settings, including use of rapid testing.

Strategy 3: Prevent new infections by working with persons diagnosed with HIV and their partners.

Strategy 4: Further decrease perinatal HIV transmission.

How Will AHP Affect Community Planning?

CPG members need to be familiar with AHP and aware of how it affects the community planning process. **As a result of the initiative, all CPGs must now select people living with HIV as the highest priority target population.** All Comprehensive HIV Prevention Plans must identify a mix of activities and interventions for these individuals because they can transmit HIV to others. As a result, focusing on improving early diagnosis and access to prevention and services for infected individuals may potentially have a large impact on reducing new infections.

These requirements do not mean that all HIV prevention resources must be used to serve people living with HIV — only that their needs must be addressed as the top priority. Your CPG will still conduct a priority setting process for other populations at high risk and your comprehensive plan will still identify a mix of interventions for those populations. However, your plan must select people living with HIV as the number one priority.

2

Roles and Responsibilities of Community Planning Participants

The key players in HIV Prevention Community Planning — health departments, CPGs, and CDC — each have individual, and in some cases shared, roles and responsibilities in the planning process. These roles and responsibilities are discussed in the following sections.

Roles and Responsibilities of CPG Members

The community planning process is complex and requires that everyone involved is carrying out their responsibilities. For that reason, it is important to lay out the specific roles and responsibilities of CPG members and give clarity to the planning tasks. This helps to avoid confusion.

As a member of the CPG, you will have a specific role to play. You may be expected to:

- Make a commitment to the planning process and its results;
- Participate in all decision making and problem-solving;
- Co-chair the process or lead a committee or workgroup;
- Serve on committees or work groups and complete assigned tasks;
- Work with the health department to gather and analyze data and other information; and
- Reflect the perspective of a specific population.

Major Responsibilities of CPGs

The major responsibilities of CPGs, and thus CPG members, are highlighted below. These responsibilities are mainly concerned with setting up the structure of the CPG, reviewing data, setting priorities, working with the health department to develop the Plan, and reviewing the health department's final funding application to CDC.

CPG Roles and Responsibilities

- Elect the community co-chair(s), this position works with the health department-designated co-chair.

- Review and use key data to establish prevention priorities.

- Develop a Comprehensive HIV Prevention Plan.

- Collaborate with the health department to review and develop key community planning products (Epidemiologic Profile, Community Services Assessment, Prioritized Populations, and Prevention Activities and Interventions).

- Review the health department application to CDC for federal HIV prevention funds, including the proposed budget. Develop a written response that describes whether the health department application does or does not, and to what degree, agree with the priorities set forth in the Comprehensive HIV Prevention Plan (Letter of Concurrence, Concurrence with Reservation, or Nonconcurrence).

- Serve as a liaison to the Communities they represent-bringing the communities' ideas and needs to the CPG and communicating the work of the CPG back to their community.

In the spirit of working collaboratively in community planning, some responsibilities are shared between CPGs and health departments. Examples of these shared responsibilities include:

- Develop procedures and policies that address membership, roles, and decision-making.

- Provide a thorough orientation for all new members as soon as possible after their appointment.

- Develop and apply criteria for selecting CPG members.

- Determine the most effective input method for the community planning process.

- Determine the amount of planning funds necessary to support community planning.

- Evaluate the planning process to ensure that it is meeting the objectives of community planning.

Length of Commitment

It is usually expected that CPG members attend regularly scheduled meetings and devote a specific number of hours each month to CPG-related activities. The length of time that you serve as a CPG member should be determined by the CPG and noted in its by-laws. Terms of service usually last at least one year and sometimes up to three years.

The CPG Co-Chair

It is important to note that one of the CPG's responsibilities is to elect one of its members to serve as the CPG's community co-chair. This person must be a member of the community and cannot be employed by the health department. The community co-chair serves alongside the health department designated co-chair to oversee the meetings and provide leadership to the group.

Terms of service vary for co-chairs and are usually defined in the CPG by-laws.

Concurrence, Concurrence with Reservations, and Nonconcurrence

One of the CPG's most important responsibilities is to review the health department's final funding application to CDC to determine whether or not the application reflects the priorities in the Plan. Based on its determination, the CPG then writes a Letter of Concurrence, Concurrence with Reservations, or Nonconcurrence to be attached to the application. Samples of all three types of letters are contained in Appendix D.

To review the three types of letters briefly:

Complete Agreement: If the CPG agrees that the health department's application reflects the Plan appropriately, then a **Letter of Concurrence** is written and submitted by the CPG.

Some Concerns: If the CPG has any concerns about the application, then a **Letter of Concurrence with Reservations** is written and submitted by the CPG. For example, the CPG may decide that the application fails to adequately address the prevention needs of a particular target population. If this is the case, then the health department must address the CPG's concerns in an attachment to the application.

No Agreement: If the CPG disagrees with most or all of the application because it does not reflect the Plan, then a **Letter of Nonconcurrence** is written and submitted by the CPG.

In cases where a health department does not agree with the CPG's recommendations in the Plan and believes that public health would be better served by funding HIV prevention activities and interventions that are substantially different, the health department must submit a letter of explanation in its application. CDC will then assess and evaluate these explanations on a case-by-case basis and determine what action may be appropriate.

When CDC receives a Letter of Nonconcurrence or Concurrence with Reservation, it may take a number of actions, including:

- Negotiating with the health department;

- Recommending local mediation;

- Conducting an on-site assessment of the situation; or

- Placing restrictions on the award of funds.

A letter of Nonconcurrence does NOT mean that your jurisdiction won't receive HIV prevention funding. It is CPG sentiment on the Plan which in turn assists in directing the CDC project officer to research further the issues related to Nonconcurrence. Samples of all three types of letters are contained in Appendix D of this Guide.

At the beginning of the planning process, it is important that CPGs develop a timeline that includes a specific amount of time for members to read the Plan, thoroughly review the health department's funding application, and discuss both documents before the health department's deadline for submitting its funding application to CDC.

SNAPSHOT OF A CPG

An Example of a Letter of Concurrence with Reservations

A CPG has reached the end of its planning cycle and has produced a Comprehensive HIV Prevention Plan. The health department has depended heavily upon the Plan in its application to CDC for HIV prevention funding. However, writing the application takes longer than expected. Finally, very close to the deadline for submitting the application, the health department brings the application to a CPG meeting, makes a brief slide presentation on the application's key points, and asks for a vote of concurrence with the application. A lively discussion takes place during which most members say they are unhappy with the timing of the application. Members want to know why they did not see it earlier. Because the submission deadline is so close, the CPG decides to attach a Letter of Concurrence with Reservations to the application. Members feel that the application is probably okay, but they have not had enough time to thoroughly review it. The health department addresses this concern in its application by explaining some of thier timeline barriers and promises to work with the CPG to develop a clear and specific timeline for the coming year. This timeline will ensure that all CPG members have ample time to review the application.

Roles and Responsibilities of Health Departments

State, local, and territorial health departments play an important role in supporting HIV Prevention Community Planning. In general, health departments provide three types of support to the community planning process: leadership, technical, and logistical.

The overall responsibilities of the health department are highlighted below:

Health Department Roles and Responsibilities

- Create and maintain at least one CPG per jurisdiction that meets the goals, objectives, and operating principles of HIV Prevention Community Planning.

- Appoint the health department co-chair.

- Keep the CPG informed of other relevant HIV prevention planning processes in the jurisdiction, and ensure collaboration between the CPG and the other efforts.

- Develop the Epidemiologic Profile and conduct the Community Services Assessment.

- Provide the CPG with information on other federal, state, and local public health services for high-risk populations identified in the Comprehensive HIV Prevention Plan.

- Ensure that CPGs have access to current HIV prevention information (including relevant budget information) and analyses of the information, including potential implications for HIV prevention in the jurisdiction.

- Develop an application to CDC for federal HIV prevention cooperative agreement funds based on the Comprehensive HIV Prevention Plan(s) developed through the HIV Prevention Community Planning process.

- Allocate, administer, and coordinate other public funds (including state, federal, and local) to prevent HIV transmission and reduce HIV-associated morbidity and mortality.

- Provide regular updates to the CPG on successes and barriers encountered in implementing the HIV prevention services described in the Comprehensive HIV Prevention Plan.

- Report progress and accomplishments to CDC.

CPG Co-Chairs and Coordinators

A health department employee is always a co-chair of the CPG, along with a community member. The health department co-chair coordinates overall planning and makes sure that the planning process is carried out effectively, involves other parts of the health department, and promotes community participation from diverse groups.

The health department co-chair is often assisted in this work by another individual, sometimes called a CPG Coordinator. The Coordinator may be a health department employee or, in some cases, an individual who is working under contract to the health department. The CPG Coordinator is often responsible for technical and logistical support to the CPG. This support may include such things as arranging meetings and meeting space, obtaining epidemiologic data, assessing community resources, disseminating materials to CPG members, and managing funds for the planning process. The Coordinator and Co-chairs may work together to develop meeting agendas and overall work plans.

Working with Other Planning Efforts in the Area

It is important for HIV prevention planning groups to be aware of other relevant planning efforts in the jurisdiction. CPGs and health departments should coordinate their HIV prevention and care planning efforts and may wish to merge HIV Prevention Community Planning with community planning for care-related services under the Ryan White Comprehensive AIDS Resources Emergency (CARE) Act.

If such mergers take place, the merged planning body is still obligated to achieve the guiding principles, goals, and objectives of the *Guidance for HIV Prevention Community Planning*.

Role and Responsibilities of CDC

Just as the health department and the CPG have roles and responsibilities to perform in the planning process, CDC also has specific roles and responsibilities related to supporting and monitoring HIV Prevention Community Planning. These are highlighted below.

CDC's Roles and Responsibilities

- Provide leadership in the national design, implementation, and evaluation of HIV Prevention Community Planning.

- Collaborate with health departments, CPGs, national organizations, federal agencies, and academic institutions to ensure that technical and program assistance and training for the community planning process are provided.

- Provide technical and program assistance through a variety of mechanisms to help recipients understand how to analyze data, prioritize target populations, identify and evaluate effective interventions, and evaluate the planning process.

- Alert health departments and CPGs about emerging trends or changes in the HIV/AIDS epidemic.

- Provide leadership in the coordination between health departments, CPGs, and directly-funded community-based organizations (CBOs).

- Monitor the HIV prevention community planning process to assist CPGs in achieving its goals and objectives.

- Collaborate with health departments in evaluating HIV prevention programs.

- Collaborate with other federal agencies and offices in promoting the transfer of new information and emerging prevention technologies or approaches to health departments and other prevention partners, including non-governmental organizations.

SNAPSHOT OF A CPG

"Okay, I think I get it. But what do I actually have to DO?"

After reading this guide, some CPG members may still say, "This is great. Lots of good information, but what do I actually have to DO?" The answer to that question will vary greatly depending on your CPG requirements and your own time, interest, and skills. Many CPGs will develop a job description for thier members. Others may just lay out basic roles and responsibilities. Most CPGs have some participation and attendance requirements for their members. These requirements should be included in the by-laws. If you are uncertain about the requirements, be sure to ask one of your CPG co-chairs. Although the require-ments may vary greatly, the basic work of a CPG member will include:

- Attending meetings and serving on Committees.

- Participating in discussions, group activities, trainings, and technical assistance.

- Sharing information based on your work or life experience.

- Reviewing information provided to you from the health department, such as the Epidemiologic Profile and Community Services Assessment.

- Talking to others in your community about their experiences and sharing that information with the CPG. Sharing the community planning experience with your community.

- Recruiting other members to the CPG, as needed.

- Gathering information, as requested, for the Community Services Assessment.

- Becoming familiar with the prioritization process.

- Participating in the consensus discussions and the implementation of the pri-ority setting process.

- Reviewing the Comprehensive HIV Prevention Plan (and in some jurisdictions helping to write it!).

- Reviewing the annual funding application submitted to CDC.

- Reviewing (or perhaps helping to draft) and signing the Letter of Concurrence, Concurrence with Reservations, or Non concurrence.

- Completing the appropriate forms to help evaluate the community planning process.

3

The Comprehensive HIV Prevention Plan and Planning Cycle

The primary task of the CPG is to develop a Comprehensive HIV Prevention Plan. The CPG is required to develop at least one plan every five years for the jurisdiction. This jurisdiction-wide plan should address all HIV prevention activities and describe how all HIV prevention funds are to be used, including federal, state, local, and when possible, private resources. The Plan must be updated every year, whether it is designed as a one-year or multi-year document.

The Key Planning Products

The Comprehensive HIV Prevention Plan consists of the key products shown in Figure 2 (see next page). The Epidemiologic Profile and the Community Services Assessment describe each of the populations most at risk of transmitting HIV or being infected, and the types of services and programs most needed by these populations. CPGs use these products to set priorities among target populations and to select interventions that will best meet the needs of each prioritized target population, as well as prevent as many new infections as possible.

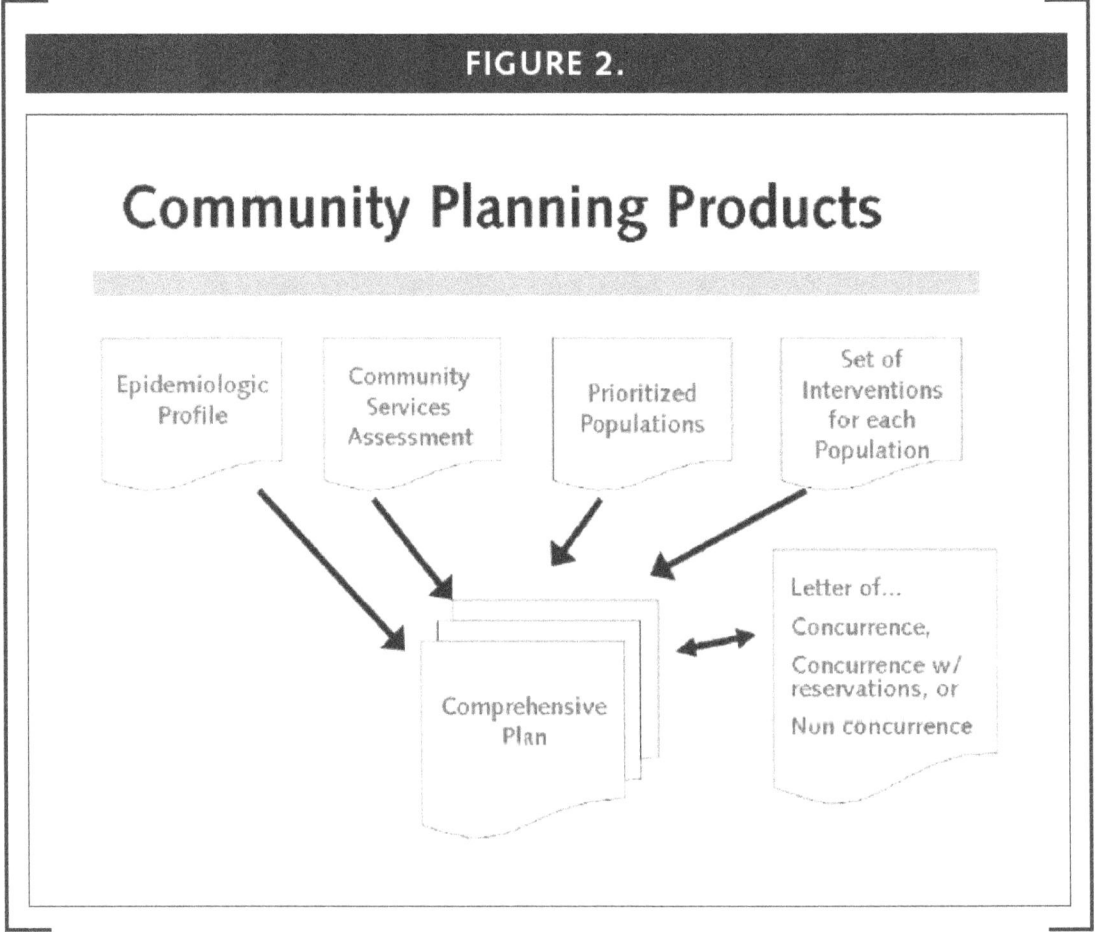

FIGURE 2.

Community Planning Products

Epidemiologic Profile

Epidemiology is the study of patterns and causes of disease and health in populations. It looks at when and where diseases are occurring, who is affected, and the risk factors that lead to disease. An Epidemiologic Profile (or "epi profile," as it is often called) features data about the impact of HIV in your community such as who is infected, who is at risk for infection, who has AIDS. Epidemiology can be very specific. For example, based on data, the epi profile documents which populations are most at risk for HIV is your community. How do we know this? Because data provide evidence of HIV transmission and behaviors associated with transmission.

The Epidemiologic Profile of local data related to HIV is vital to the CPG's work because it provides the basis for defining target populations.

Collaborating in the Development of Epi Profiles

In preparing the epi profile, the HIV Prevention Community Planning Group should work with their state or local Ryan White CARE Act planning group to develop one integrated profile for use by both groups. A document called *Integrated Guidelines for Developing Epidemiologic Profiles: HIV Prevention and Ryan White CARE Act Community Planning* is available to review and download at: **www.cdc.gov/hiv/pubs/epi_guide/epi_guidelines.pdf** or at **www.hivaidsta.org**.

These guidelines were developed by CDC and the Health Resources and Services Administration (HRSA) to help health departments produce integrated epi profiles and to advise them on how to interpret data in ways that are consistent and useful for HIV prevention and CARE planning groups.

Community Services Assessment

The community services assessment (CSA) is a process of gathering information about:

- The prevention needs of populations at risk of HIV infection (Needs Assesment)

- The prevention activities and interventions currently being carried out to address these needs (Resource Inventory)

- Any existing gaps in services (Gap Analysis)

The CSA includes a mix of qualitative and quantitative information that might be obtained from surveys, focus groups, interviews or other ways of gathering information from affected and infected populations. **The CSA provides context for setting HIV prevention priorities. The findings should feed into the CPG's decision-making process, including priority setting.**

A guide to assessing needs was developed by (AED) the Academy for Educational Development and may be useful to CPGs. *Assessing the Need for HIV Prevention Services: A Guide for Community Planning Groups* can be accessed at **www.hivaidsta.org**.

Prioritized Target Populations

The Comprehensive HIV Prevention Plan must include a set of prioritized target populations who need prevention services. Populations are prioritized by comparing infection rates, risk behaviors, and other factors. This process helps health departments direct prevention funds to those populations most at risk of transmitting HIV or becoming infected. As a result, targeted prevention efforts can be supported to reduce HIV transmission in populations with the highest rates of HIV infection, thereby achieving the greatest impact possible. **Remember, under CDC's Advancing HIV Prevention initiative, CPGs are now required to make people living with HIV the highest priority population. This is because of their risk of transmitting HIV to others, especially those who are infected but who do not know it.**

A guide to setting HIV prevention priorities that may be useful to CPGs was developed by AED. *Setting HIV Prevention Priorities: A Guide for Community Planning Groups* may be accessed at **www.hivaidsta.org**.

Appropriate Science-Based Prevention Activities and Interventions

The Comprehensive HIV Prevention Plan must contain recommendations for a mix of prevention activities and interventions that are science-based and appropriate for each prioritized target population.

"Science-based" means that proposed activities and interventions must be ones that research or theory have proven to be effective. Such interventions are now being disseminated throughout the U.S. by CDC. CPGs are encouraged to use them if they are right for their locality and target populations. "Appropriate" means that proposed activities and interventions must fit the culture and ethnicity of target populations and respond to their specific needs.

The Community Planning Cycle

The planning cycle is the period of time during which a CPG completes its products and develops a comprehensive plan. The community planning process should be flexible, so the *Guidance* allows for a planning cycle to cover a one- to five-year period. It is important that health departments and CPGs decide jointly what their approach to the planning process will be, the steps that will be involved in carrying out all necessary processes and products, and a reasonable timeline (or planning cycle) for the planning process. CPGs may choose from the following options:

Key Milestones in the Planning Cycle

- Complete each planning product

- Conduct an annual review of the plan

- Update the plan

- Decide whether to concur, concur with reservations, or not concur with the health department funding application

- Health department submits funding application to CDC

■ A CPG may choose to complete the planning process and submit a plan in one year. In this case, each community planning product must be completed every year.

■ A CPG may choose to complete the entire planning process over a two-year period. In the first year, while it is beginning its two-year planning process, the CPG is required to update its most recent Comprehensive HIV Prevention Plan and complete a concurrence process. In year two, the CPG develops a new plan and carries out the concurrence process. The CPG would then have two years to carry out the CSA and conduct a prioritization process.

■ A CPG may choose to complete the planning process over three, four, or five years. In this case, the CPG would need to either update the most recent plan and complete a concurrence process, or develop a new plan and complete a concurrence process each year, depending on the length of the cycle.

HIV Prevention Community Planning: An Orientation Guide

4

Group Process

Like any group process, community planning needs to be set up in a way that decreases confusion or conflict and makes getting the work done easier. This means that CPGs should discuss and put in writing how they will conduct their business, make decisions, handle conflict, and complete day-to-day activities. This section addresses some ways to ensure a smooth process.

If you are joining an established CPG, policies for conducting business will probably already be in place. However, it may be useful for you to see the types of questions that were involved in initially creating these process policies. They also will be useful if your CPG decides to revisit or revise its policies.

By-laws

By-laws are the CPG's written rules of operation. They are written down as a reference because they provide the framework and often the "final word" on how the CPG will do business. By-laws should cover at least the following issues. The issues are stated as questions that CPGs should ask themselves in order to clarify how things will be done.

- What is the purpose or mission of the CPG?

- How will the CPG be directed? Will it choose to have officers such as committee chairs, a secretary, or others? How are these leaders selected? What are their roles and responsibilities? When will their terms expire?

- How often does the CPG meet? What is the composition of the CPG?

- By what process are CPG members recruited and selected? What are the criteria for being a member? How long do members serve? Can a member be removed for any reason? If so, how is this done?

- What are the roles and responsibilities of CPG members? Will committees be used? If so, which committees will be used? What are the roles of these committees?

- What happens when a conflict occurs? By what process does the CPG resolve conflicts? Are conflicts and resolutions documented?

- What is the CPG's policy on conflict(s) of interest?

- By what process can the by-laws be changed?

Ground Rules

Ground rules are usually less formal than by-laws although they should always be written down. Ground rules are the CPG's collective thinking about how members are going to get along with each other most effectively while working together.

Each CPG should establish its own ground rules. For the rules to be effective, all members must agree with them and abide by them. Some CPGs find it helpful to post the ground rules at each meeting for easy reference and reminder.

Sample Ground Rules

- Show mutual respect during and outside meetings.

- Only one person talks at a time.

- Keep the CPG's internal discussions confidential ("What's said here stays here"), unless confidentiality is not appropriate or required.

- Respect individual roles and responsibilities.

- Perform assigned duties and tasks on time and as completely as possible.

- Turn off, and do not talk on, cell phones during meetings.

- Begin and end meetings on time.

Conflicts of Interest

A conflict of interest (COI) can be defined as a conflict between one's obligation to the public good and one's self interest. In community planning, a COI may occur when a member knowingly takes action to influence the CPG in order to gain financial or other benefit for themselves, their family, or their agency.

Conflicts of interest can occur when CPG members who are advocates for a particular group or associated with a certain organization participate in a process that needs to meet the needs of many groups. For example, a CPG member who works primarily in HIV prevention with drug users is likely to advocate for issues affecting drug users. Although this is unavoidable and is often desirable, the CPG member must be able to participate objectively (without bias and based on data) in a priority setting process that gives fair and equal consideration to all populations. The situation can be difficult if the CPG member's agency or position is affected by the CPG's decisions.

To deal with potential conflicts of interest, CPGs should develop a **Conflict of Interest Statement** that gives clear guidance on how to handle these situations. The policies may vary from group to group and can include a variety of actions, including barring participation in discussion and/or votes on the specific issues related to the conflict. At a minimum, CPG members should always disclose potential conflicts or relationships that might result in a conflict before participating in decision making. **It is vital to deal with any conflict of interest BEFORE beginning the priority setting process.**

SNAPSHOT OF A CPG

Using By-Laws and Conflict of Interest Statements

A CPG has reached the point where target populations are to be prioritized. One member points out that at least two other members have a conflict of interest. Both of these CPG members are employees of agencies that may gain financially, depending on what populations are prioritized. The question the CPG needs to answer is: Should these members be allowed to participate in priority setting? The CPG co-chair reminds everyone that they have all signed conflict of interest statements and that the by-laws contain detailed policies on this subject. A portion of the meeting is set aside to review the by-laws and the CPG's Conflict of Interest Statement. Based on this CPG's policies, the members in question are allowed to participate in the discussion and the priority setting process, but must refrain from participating in any voting relating to the populations they serve. Because this CPG had already developed clear by-laws and Conflict of Interest Statements, the group is able to move forward with their important community planning work without further delay.

Decision Making

In the course of a planning cycle, CPGs must make many decisions. As a result, CPGs need to decide how they are going to make decisions as a group. The following questions may help focus this discussion.

- What is the process for making decisions?

- Who makes which decisions?

- Can some decisions be made by individuals without group approval? If so, which decisions and who makes them?

- Should the CPG have a written policy for making decisions?

- When is a decision final?

- Are some decisions out of the CPG's hands? If so, which decisions are these? If a member does not agree with a decision, is there a process for challenging or appealing it?

A CPG can use many approaches to come to group decisions, including consensus, simple majority vote or other methods for making choices. Some CPGs have adapted or modified Robert's Rules of Order as a way of running meetings and making decisions. The most important factor is that every member of the CPG clearly understands and agrees to the method of decision making.

Committees

CPGs often use committees to do much of the work of community planning. Committees can examine issues and develop recommendations more efficiently and effectively than the group as a whole. Some committees may have written policies or rules of operation. Most will have a chairperson who reports to the CPG co-chairs.

Committees are particularly useful for discrete tasks, such as recruiting and selecting new members, or completing tasks that take place over a defined time during a planning cycle, such as determing priority populations or prevention interventions. CPGs also often have standing committees, which exist permanently, not just for completing a specific task. An example is an Executive Committee, which provides continuing leadership and management support to the CPG.

No committee actually does **all** of the work itself. They will, however, be responsible for doing the ground work and preparing recommendations for the entire CPG. This division of labor ensures that the work gets done by the CPG, but individual members don't get overburdened or

4

overwhelmed. The small group, or committee, approach also makes it easier to collect information and develop recommendations.

CPG members should learn the committee structure for their CPG and participate on one or more committees.

SNAPSHOT OF A CPG

Based on discussions among all members, a statewide CPG decides to form three separate committees as an effective and efficient means to complete its work. These three committees are: (1) the Community Services Assessment committee, (2) the priority populations committee, and (3) the interventions committee. Each committee has a defined scope of work and clear roles and responsibilities for its members. Each CPG member must serve on **ONE** of the committees. Early in the planning cycle, the CSA committee will be busiest. They will work with the health department to determine a CSA process and may assist in gathering information and analyzing the findings. When this committee has finished its work, the priority populations committee gets busy developing a prioritization process and determining the best use for the assessment data. At the same time, the interventions committee may begin gathering information on effective interventions and preparing to identify a set of interventions for the rank-ordered priority populations.

Conflict Resolution

Not all decision making involves conflict, but sometimes conflict is a necessary part of making good decisions. CPGs need to determine how and by whom conflicts will be resolved. What happens, for example, if members sharply disagree about priority target populations or the mix of interventions proposed in the Plan? Or if they cannot come to an agreement about group process?

Conflict can be dealt with in many ways, and the most effective method depends on the nature of the group and the nature of the conflict. For some disputes, groups may choose to use a formal mediation process in which a conflict is put into writing and an outside individual attempts to resolve the conflict. In other situations, the best method is a process in which a special committee of disinterested individuals is appointed to deal with the conflict. **CPGs should decide on some formal process for resolving conflicts — before any disagreements arise, if possible.**

Facilitation

Many groups use facilitators to help members get through their discussions efficiently and make decisions effectively. Facilitators create an environment in which group members can share ideas, opinions, experiences, and expertise to achieve a common goal. A skilled facilitator can smooth the way for group members to discuss issues, brainstorm options, and identify viable solutions. A skilled facilitator is also sensitive to diverse cultures and communication styles. The facilitator can help elicit input and participation from individuals who might otherwise be overlooked.

Effective facilitation of meetings is important because it provides a structure for the process, keeps the meetings focused, helps to keep good order and assists members in addressing agenda items and any issues that may arise. Effective facilitation can also help to prevent or resolve conflicts that may arise during meetings.

Like other groups who deal with complex issues, CPG members benefit from facilitation. Often, one or both of the co-chairs facilitate the meetings. However, some CPGs choose to enlist the services of an outside professional to facilitate their meetings.

A guide is available from AED — *Facilitating Meetings: A Guide for Community Planning Groups* — that may useful to CPGs. You can access this guide at **www.hivaidsta.org**.

5

Monitoring and Evaluating the Community Planning Process

Monitoring and evaluating HIV Prevention Community Planning is a shared responsibility of the health department and the CPG. However, health departments are ultimately responsible for reporting monitoring and evaluation activities to CDC.

Goals, Objectives, and Attributes

Community planning monitoring and evaluating activities are based on the three goals and eight objectives described in chapter 1. Each goal provides an overall direction for community planning. Because the goals are broad, the objectives define specific processes and products that are needed to achieve each goal. In addition, 52 critical attributes have been defined to measure the implementation and achievement of objectives (see Appendix E).

This structure for monitoring and evaluating community planning may seem complicated but it's actually straightforward and will help CPGs do their job well. It works like this:

- CPGs have some broad tasks they need to accomplish (**goals**).

- To accomplish these broad tasks, certain specific processes and products need to be developed (**objectives**).

- Achieving the objectives is complex and involves very detailed work (**attributes**). The attributes are key. They provide a detailed "roadmap" of what needs to happen throughout the planning process.

The figure below illustrates how goals, objectives and attributes work together.

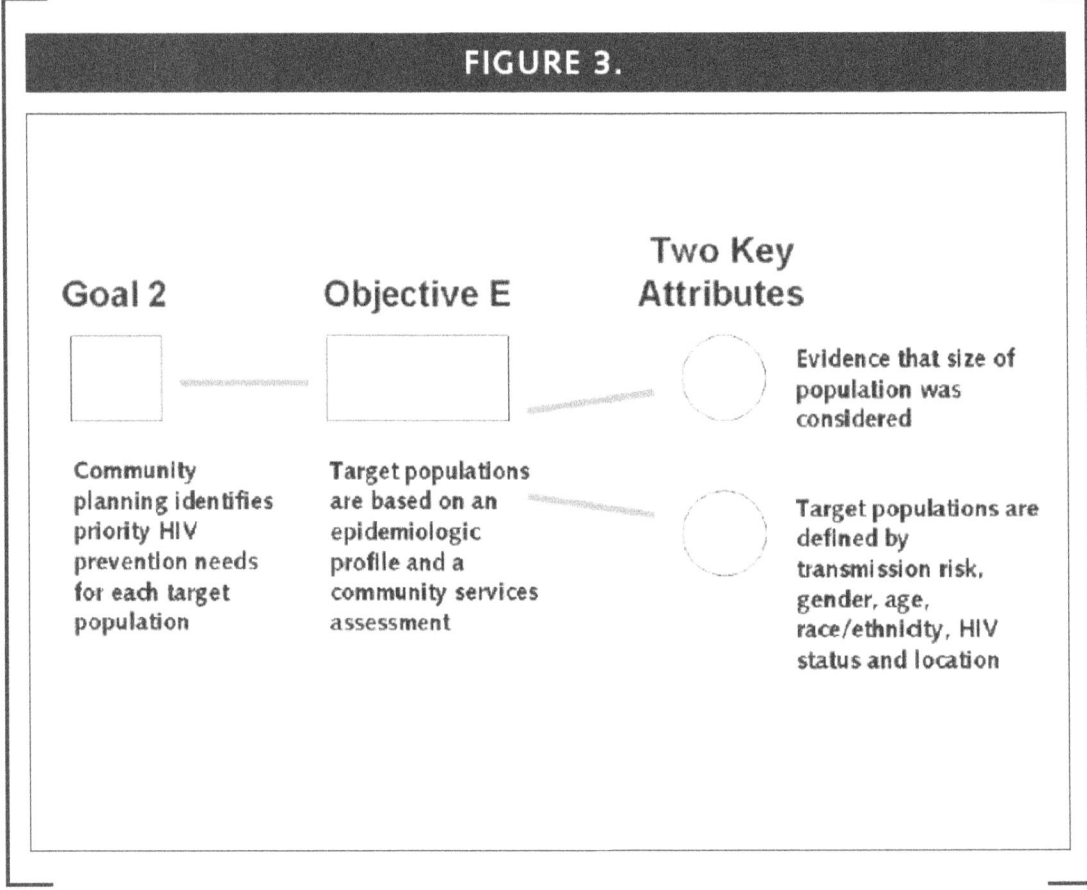

FIGURE 3.

Goal 2

Community planning identifies priority HIV prevention needs for each target population

Objective E

Target populations are based on an epidemiologic profile and a community services assessment

Two Key Attributes

Evidence that size of population was considered

Target populations are defined by transmission risk, gender, age, race/ethnicity, HIV status and location

If the attributes for a particular objective are present in the planning process, then a CPG can know with some confidence that the objective is being met. If the objectives for each goal are being met, then that goal is most likely being achieved.

The box below, which contains one objective of the planning process and its associated attributes, is a good way to demonstrate the importance of the attributes in monitoring the planning process. As you review the attributes, note how each one provides specific guidance to the CPG about what needs to happen to achieve the planning objective.

> *Planning Objective E: To ensure that priority target populations are based on an epidemiologic profile and a community services assessment. The presence of the following attributes is critical to achieving this objective:*
>
> - **Attribute 37:** Evidence that the size of at-risk populations was considered in setting priorities for target populations.
>
> - **Attribute 38:** Evidence that a measurement of the percentage of HIV morbidity (i.e., HIV/AIDS incidence or prevalence), if available, was considered in setting priorities for target populations.
>
> - **Attribute 39:** Evidence that the prevalence of risky behaviors in the population was considered in setting priorities for target populations.
>
> - **Attribute 40:** Target populations are defined by transmission risk, gender, age, race/ethnicity, HIV status, and geographic location.
>
> - **Attribute 41:** Target populations are rank ordered by priority, in terms of their contribution to new HIV infections.

Program Performance Indicators

In addition to monitoring the planning goals, objectives, and attributes, health departments are responsible for monitoring program performance indicators and reporting them to CDC through the Program Evaluation Monitoring System (PEMS). Program performance indicators provide information about how well a CPG is doing in carrying out its community planning responsibilities. It measures a CPG's progress in meeting the goals and objectives of community planning. Performance indicators assist CDC in tracking work produced and results achieved. There are four indicators for community planning, which focus on:

- The community planning process;

- Community planning membership;

- Linkages between the priorities in the Plan and the health department application to CDC; and

- Linkages between the priorities in the Plan and the actual funded interventions

The specific indicators are:

Indicator E.1: The proportion of populations most at risk, as documented in the epidemiologic profile, that have at least one CPG member who reflects the perspective of each population. In other words, does the CPG include members who reflect each of the populations identified as most at risk for HIV in that jurisdiction?

Indicator E.2: The proportion of key attributes of an HIV Prevention Community Planning process that CPG members agree has occurred. In other words, is the CPG effectively achieving the specific tasks, activities, or processes (represented by the attributes) for each of its planning objectives?

Indicator E.3: The percent of prevention interventions and supporting activities in the health department's CDC funding application specified as a priority in the Comprehensive HIV Prevention Plan. In other words, how accurately does the funding application reflect the Plan?

Indicator E.4: The percent of health department-funded prevention interventions and supporting activities that correspond to priorities specified in the Comprehensive HIV Prevention Plan. In other words, how accurately do the interventions actually funded by the health department reflect intervention priorities in the Plan?

Appendix F contains two tools that are used to measure these indicators — the *HIV Prevention Community Planning Membership Survey* and the *Community Planning Linkage Table Worksheet*.

How Do Monitoring and Evaluation Tools Measure the Indicators?

CPG members are asked to complete the *Community Planning Membership Survey*. The survey contains many questions designed to get each CPG member's perspective on how the community planning process works in their jurisdiction. It also asks CPG members whether the objectives for community planning have been met during the most recent year of planning. This is measured using the key attributes. The information from this survey helps the health department measure the first two indicators and will be reported to CDC.

- The first indicator requires CPG members to compare their Epidemiologic Profile with their *Membership Survey* and asks, "How many populations most at risk for HIV are represented by at least one CPG member?"

- The second indicator asks CPG members to look at all responses to the *Membership Survey* and determine, "Based on CPG members' agreement, how many attributes have occurred or been addressed, this year?"

The other two performance indicators for community planning are measured through the use of a document called the *Linkages Table Worksheet*. These tables are completed by the health department. However, the health department will need to base its answers on the work of the CPG.

- The third indicator asks the health department, "How many of the interventions/activities in your application were specified as a priority in the Comprehensive HIV Prevention Plan?"

- The fourth indicator asks the health department, "How many of the interventions/activities funded by the health department match up with the priorities in the Comprehensive HIV Prevention Plan?"

Roles and Responsibilities in Monitoring and Evaluation

Although all the partners work together to monitor and evaluate the activities of a CPG and its results, each partner has specific roles and responsibilities:

Health Departments

Health departments bear the primary responsibility for tracking whether or not planning goals, objectives, and attributes are being achieved. They are responsible for reporting monitoring and evaluation data to CDC through PEMS.

Community Planning Groups

CPG members play a crucial role in monitoring the planning process by ensuring that the goals and objectives of community planning are met. By doing so, CPG members ensure an effective planning process and provide accountability to CDC for their planning activities.

CPG members fulfill this monitoring and accountability role by working with the health department to assess whether the community planning program performance indicators are present in the planning process. CPG members should be familiar with the program performance indicators for community planning and the criteria for monitoring them.

CDC

CDC is responsible for providing leadership in the evaluation of community planning and for providing evaluation technical assistance to health departments to promote more effective evaluation of community planning.

CDC's *Evaluating CDC-funded Health Department HIV Prevention Programs* contains a wealth of useful information about monitoring and evaluating the community planning process, including details on:

- Conducting the *Community Planning Membership Survey;*
- Describing priority populations;
- Describing a set of prevention interventions and activities; and
- Assessing the linkages between the Comprehensive HIV Prevention Plan and CDC funding application, as well as linkages between the Plan and funded interventions.

This document can be found at: www.cdc.gov/hiv/aboutdhap/perb/hdg.htm.

6

Technical Assistance in HIV Prevention Community Planning

A time usually comes when CPG members need help to do their planning work more effectively. This help is called technical assistance (TA), or Capacity Building Assistance (CBA). TA/CBA is available in a variety of forms and in a number of subject areas, and it's only a phone call away. The assistance may involve:

- Helping a CPG assess when assistance might be needed

- Arranging for peers to share common experiences and to brainstorm ideas

- Improving access for, and participation of, infected and affected populations in the planning process

- Providing a specific skills training for CPG members (for example, priority setting)

- Assisting the CPG in dealing with group process issues or conflict resolution

- Working with a CPG subcommittee on specific processes

Who Now Comprises the TA Network?

CDC supports eight organizations — the **National TA Providers Network** — to provide TA to CPGs. The network providers work together to:

- Identify and clarify TA needs

- Identify local, regional, and/or national TA providers and peers

- Arrange for providers to deliver TA

- Monitor the delivery and effectiveness of TA

- Develop tools for use by CPGs and health departments to support community planning

Partners in the National TA Providers' Network include:

- Academy for Educational Development (AED)

- Asian and Pacific Islander American Health Forum (APIAHF)

- Behavioral and Social Science Volunteer (BSSV) Program, American Psychological Association

- Inter Tribal Council of Arizona, Inc. (ITCA)

- National AIDS Education & Services for Minorities (NAESM)

- National Alliance of State and Territorial AIDS Directors (NASTAD)

- National Association of People with AIDS (NAPWA)

- U.S.-Mexico Border Health Association (USMBHA)

The TA/CBA Process

In What Ways Can CPGs Receive TA/CBA?

CDC has developed a CBA Request Tracking System. This system is a reactive process designed to respond to and track individual capacity building assistance requests from CBA consumers. To access the system, a CPG must first contact their CDC Project Officer to make the request. Your Project Officer will work with the CDC CBA Coordinator to identify the appropriate TA/CBA provider. The TA/CBA provider will work with you to identify the TA/CBA approach and delivery method. TA/CBA may be delivered in several ways, including:

- Holding telephone conversations

- Giving CPGs information and self-help materials

- Reviewing materials

- Conducting on-site visits to discuss issues and approaches, assist in developing methods or processes or conduct workshops or specific training sessions

- Referring CPGs to specific TA sources or materials

When Is It Time to Seek Help?

CPGs should ask for help when they experience difficulty with a specific planning task or process. For example, a CPG might need help with monitoring and evaluation or priority setting. A CPG might also request technical assistance as it begins developing or implementing a new process. CPGs might also ask for technical assistance if they encounter challenges or conflicts among members.

How Do CPGs Request Help?

Requesting TA involves a few easy steps:

- Begin by asking, "What types of knowledge, skills, or support do we need to accomplish our planning tasks or objectives?" The CPG should discuss these issues **before** making a TA/CBA request.

  For example, during the planning process, conflicts may arise within the CPG. Ask yourselves these questions:

  - *Do we understand how to manage or respond to conflict?*

  - *Do we have the skills necessary to manage conflict? What are those skills?*

  - *What support are we receiving to manage conflict, and is that support helpful?*

  Another example concerns task-related activities, such as prioritizing target populations. When you get to priority setting, you may find that it's more difficult than you thought. Ask yourselves these questions:

  - *Do we understand how to prioritize target populations? What do we need to do?*

  - *Do we have the data analysis or other skills needed to prioritize populations? What skills do we need? Do we have all or just some of those skills?*

  - *What support are we receiving to prioritize populations, and is that support helpful?*

- The health department, CPG co-chairs, and other CPG members should all contribute to the TA request. All members of the CPG should discuss and agree on the expected outcomes of TA/CBA and the commitment necessary for the TA to happen effectively.

- The CPG should designate one person as the "point of contact" for coordinating TA/CBA. The contact person serves as a liaison between the CPG and the provider, scheduling calls, communicating with members, and arranging the actual TA/CBA delivery.

- The CPG should contact its CDC Project Officer. CDC will work with the CPG co-chairs or point of contact person, the CPG, and the TA/CBA provider to develop a specific plan to meet your TA needs.

In What Subject Areas Is TA/CBA Available?

TA/CBA is always tailored to a CPG's specific needs, so the following list of TA subject areas may or may not be relevant to your situation. In the past, TA has often been requested in these areas:

- **Orientation to the Community Planning Process**
  May include TA/CBA on: what planning group members should know about community planning; identifying the community planning components; and understanding roles and responsibilities and the expected outcome of community planning.

- **Process Management**
  May include TA/CBA on: managing member nomination and selection; setting ground rules; managing conflict; conducting effective meetings; establishing a decision making process; and collaborating with other planning efforts.

- **Parity, Inclusion and Representation (PIR)**
  May include TA/CBA on: identifying and involving a variety of individuals, communities, organizations, professionals, and affected groups; improving the capacity of members to represent their communities; and enhancing cultural diversity and improving cultural competency.

- **Using Data to Support Decision making**
  May include TA/CBA on: understanding the epidemiologic profile; using epidemiologic information; increasing familiarity with data sources and their strengths and limitations.

- **Community Services Assessment**
  May include TA/CBA on: using different assessment strategies (e.g., surveys, evaluation findings, focus groups, public meetings); developing a description of HIV prevention resources; comparing the need with the resources to develop a gap analysis; and merging a Community Services Assessment process with the Ryan White assessment process.

- **Priority setting**
  May include TA/CBA on: setting priorities among target populations; identifying and selecting interventions; and using effective group decision making.

- **Intervention Effectiveness ("What Works")**
  May include TA/CBA on: objectively examining intervention effectiveness; and gain a basic understanding of behavioral science for HIV prevention.

- **Evaluation of the Planning Process**
  May include TA/CBA on: understanding the key attributes of community planning and the Community Planning Membership Survey; monitoring and documenting progress; and assessing the development and implementation of the HIV prevention plan.

7

Customizing Your Orientation Guide

We've noticed that many CPG members add tabs at the back of guides like this to include important information about their own CPGs and planning process. We've added this section to allow you to do just that. Appendix G contains additional resources you may also find helpful.

Though you'll make your own decisions about what to include in this section, we suggest you consider the following items that are specific to your CPG and planning process:

- Mission statement

- By-laws

- Committee or subcommittee structure and staffing

- Ground rules

- Meeting minutes

- Decision-making process and procedures

- Job descriptions (example: co-chairs, subcommittee chairs, etc.)

- Timeline, work plan, calendar, or planning cycle

- CPG member contact information

- Common abbreviations, acronyms, and glossary of terms

- Conflict of interest statement

Appendices

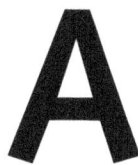

A

Community Planning Orientation Self-Assessment Checklist

Now that you have read the *HIV Prevention Community Planning: An Orientation Guide* and the *Guidance for HIV Prevention Community Planning*, you should be fairly familiar with the HIV prevention community planning process. You may have already participated in an orientation with your CPG.

This checklist can serve as a self assessment tool to see how much you have learned and what questions you may still have. Check the box for each statement you believe is true. For those boxes you have not checked, make a list of questions and arrange a time to meet with one of your co-chairs to have your questions answered.

☐ I know the name of my HIV Prevention Community Planning Group (CPG).

☐ I can name the co-chairs of our CPG.

☐ I know who is responsible for HIV Prevention Community Planning at our state or local health department.

☐ I understand what the Comprehensive HIV Prevention Plan is.

☐ I understand the difference between the Comprehensive HIV Prevention Plan and the application to CDC.

☐ I know what PIR stands for and what it means.

☐ I know what an Epidemiologic Profile (epi profile) is.

☐ I know what a Community Services Assessment (CSA) is.

☐ I understand how our CPG conducts the CSA.

☐ I know what it means to prioritize populations.

☐ I can name my jurisdiction's priority populations.

☐ I understand the different types of prevention interventions and activities for various populations.

☐ I understand our CPGs prioritization process.

☐ I have my own copy of the 2004-2008 *Guidance for HIV Prevention Community Planning*.

☐ I understand my job on our CPG.

☐ I have a copy of our CPG's by-laws.

☐ I have seen and understand our CPG's ground rules.

☐ I understand how our CPG makes decisions.

☐ I understand how our CPG conducts meetings.

☐ I can name our CPGs committees.

☐ I know which committee(s) I want to participate on.

☐ I have seen and understand our CPG's work plan and timeline.

☐ I understand the Letter of Concurrence, Concurrence with Reservations or Non-Concurrence.

☐ I have seen and signed our CPG's Conflict of Interest Statement.

☐ I know the length of my term as a CPG member.

☐ I know how our CPG recruits new members.

☐ I know who our CDC Project Officer is.

☐ I know which population or community I represent on the CPG and how to be a voice for them in the community planning process.

☐ I know what to do and who to approach if I have a problem or a grievance.

☐ Yo sé donde puedo encontrar información en Espanol si lo necesito / I know where I can get information available in Spanish if I need it.

☐ I know to request technical assistance (TA)

B

Summary of Changes in the 2004-2008 *Guidance for HIV Prevention Community Planning*

With the revision of the *Guidance for HIV Prevention Community Planning* in 2003, several changes have taken place in the community planning process. The following table summarizes those changes:

SUMMARY OF THE *GUIDANCE*: THEN (1998) AND NOW (2004-2008)		
ISSUE	**THEN**	**NOW**
Principles	The *Guidance* had 15 guiding principles.	The *Guidance* has 10 guiding principles. Principles with similar themes or ideas were revised and combined.
Goal and Objectives	The *Guidance* had five core objectives.	The former objectives have been changed to three broader goals. Each goal now has either two or three corresponding objectives, for a total of eight objectives.
Steps/Products	The *Guidance* specified nine steps in developing the Plan.	The nine steps CPGs were using have been taken out of the *Guidance*. The current *Guidance* focuses on the planning process and key products. As before, the major product for the planning cycle is the Comprehensive HIV Prevention Plan. *Note: Although the steps are not delineated, CPGs will still accomplish the same core activities in completing key products.*

SUMMARY OF THE *GUIDANCE*: THEN (1998) AND NOW (2004-2008)

ISSUE	THEN	NOW
Roles and Responsibilities	Roles and responsibilities were defined for CPG members, health departments, and CDC.	The roles and responsibilities detailed in the former version of the *Guidance* have been updated and revised.
People Living with HIV	CPGs often prioritized people living with HIV as a priority population.	CPGs must now prioritize people living with HIV as the number one priority population.
Community Services Assessment (CSA)	The needs assessment, the gap analysis and the resource inventory were three separate processes.	The *Guidance* now defines these processes as a Community Services Assessment. Responsibility for implementing the CSA is now primarily the role of the health department with input and review from CPGs.
Priority Setting	CPGs were required to rank and prioritize populations and interventions for each population.	CPGs still prioritize populations, but no longer have to prioritize interventions. Instead, CPGs will identify a set of interventions for each population.
Evaluation	Evaluation of the community planning process was a vital process.	The *Guidance* now contains a section on Monitoring and Evaluation, including concrete measures of progress and tools to help CPGs monitor and evaluate progress toward meeting the objectives.
Appendices	The *Guidance* did not contain appendices.	The *Guidance* contains several user-friendly appendices, including: • A sample conflict of interest statement • Sample letters of Concurrence, Concurrence with Reservation and Nonconcurrence • The HIV Prevention Community Planning Attributes • A glossary
External Review	The *Guidance* required external review of the Plan, a process through which outside panels of people reviewed Comprehensive HIV Prevention Plans from several localities.	External review has been eliminated. CDC Project Officers will continue to do technical reviews of health department applications for funding, which are based on the comprehensive plans. The addition of tools for monitoring and evaluation in the *Guidance* will help CDC track the progress of CPGs toward meeting their objectives.

C

Putting the "P" in PIR: Tips for Orienting Your CPG

You are probably familiar with the commonly used term "PIR." As the cornerstone of community planning, PIR is referenced regularly. Although most CPGs do a good job of ensuring **inclusion**, **representation** of affected populations is often more difficult, and many groups struggle to address the **parity** piece of the equation.

Parity means that all members can equally participate and carry out the community planning tasks. This means that each member understands the community planning process and their own individual roles and responsibilities.

Key Issues for Orienting your CPG

One of the primary ways to achieve parity is to ensure that all members have a solid foundation in the basics of community planning. This foundation can be achieved by having all members participate in an orientation to HIV prevention community planning. Although your CPG's orientation should be tailored to meet the specific needs of your members, the following questions should be addressed by any orientation for new members.

- What is HIV prevention community planning?
  - What is the history of community planning in general?
  - What is the history of community planning in our jurisdiction?
  - Why do we do local community planning?
  - Who participates on a CPG?
  - What is PIR?
- What is the *Guidance for HIV Prevention Community Planning*?

- ■ What products do health departments and CPGs develop?
  - • Epidemiologic Profile
  - • Community Services Assessment
  - • Prioritization of Populations
  - • Identification of Interventions
  - • "The Plan"
  - • "The Application"
  - • Letter of Concurrence, Concurrence with Reservations or Non-Concurrence
- ■ What is a Comprehensive HIV Prevention Plan?
- ■ What does it mean to "prioritize populations?"
- ■ How does community planning work in our jurisdiction?
  - • When do we meet?
  - • Who participates on our CPG?
  - • Do we have committees?
  - • How long is our planning cycle?
  - • What does it mean to be a member of our CPG?
  - • Who are our co-chairs?
  - • Do we have a timeline and workplan for completing our tasks?
- ■ What are by-laws and what do ours say?
- ■ How does our CPG make decisions?
- ■ How does our CPG handle conflict?
- ■ How does our CPG handle conflict of interest?
- ■ How does our CPG ensure PIR?
- ■ What is the role of our health department?
- ■ What is the role of CDC?
- ■ What is my role as a CPG member?
- ■ What are our priorities?
  - • How have these priorities been implemented in our jurisdiction?
- ■ What are the ground rules for our meetings?
- ■ How do we evaluate out community planning process?
- ■ How are CPG members involved in monitoring and evaluating community planning?

An orientation to community planning is vital for new members who need to understand the community planning process, but it can also be a useful experience for more seasoned members. An orientation provides an opportunity to refresh knowledge and skills. It is also a chance to talk about updates, new information, or changes in the process. Many CPGs ask their seasoned members to provide support in implementing and delivering the orientation.

Ask your AED Technical Assistance Liaison or CDC Project Officer for additional resources that can help you develop your own orientation to HIV Prevention Community Planning. You can also access materials and resources at www.hivaidsta.org.

How often should our CPG provide an Orientation?

The answer to this question will vary from one jurisdiction to another. Your CPG should decide based on a variety of factors including:

- Frequency of member turnover;

- Frequency of your meetings;

- Number of new members; and

- Availability of staff, materials, and resources

Some CPGs choose to offer an orientation once or twice a year. Other CPGs offer individual orientations every time they get a new member. Sometimes CPGs will combine an orientation with an annual retreat. While others will do some portion of the orientation at each meeting to ensure ongoing skill building and information exchange.

Some CPGs have implemented a "buddy" or "mentoring" system in which more experienced members will work with new members to share information, answer questions, and provide support as they learn about the process.

C

D

Sample Letters of Concurrence, Concurrence with Reservations, and Nonconcurrence

Sample Letters of Concurrence, Concurrence with Reservations or Nonconcurrence

SAMPLE 1 - Statewide Community Planning Group: *LETTER OF CONCURRENCE*

Date

Mr./Ms._____

Grants Management Officer

Procurement and Grants Office

Centers for Disease Control and Prevention

290 Brandywine Road

Room 300, Mailstop E-15

Atlanta, GA 30341

Dear Mr./Ms._____ :

The_____HIV community planning group confirmed by consensus at its meeting August 8-9, 2003, its concurrence with the state of _____'s application to CDC for HIV prevention funds under program announcement 04012. The planning group has reviewed the state's proposed 2004 objectives, activities, and budget and finds them to be responsive to the priorities identified by the planning group and expressed in the _____ HIV prevention plan, 2003-2005.

The planning group met _____ (frequency) during 2003 and through a series of full-group and subcommittee meetings planned the content of meetings, defined needs established in the existing plan, and developed a schedule to review the state's HIV prevention application. Members were asked to review materials (the HIV prevention plan 2003-2005 and the state's 2004 AIDS/STD program plan objectives) and be prepared to discuss them at the September meeting. Thirteen of the 16 planning group members reviewed progress on the state's 2003 objectives, the planning group priorities, the HIV prevention plan 2003-2005, and the state's draft 2004 program plan and objectives. At the August planning group meeting, members gave AIDS/STD program staff considerable feedback on content for the 2004 CDC application. Based on a review of the draft program plan, the planning group easily reached consensus on its concurrence that the priorities and strategies proposed for the state's application reflected the priorities expressed in the planning group's plan.

The two community co-chairs, along with the health department co-chair, have been designated as signatories to the letter of concurrence.

Sincerely,

2004–2008 HIV PREVENTION COMMUNITY PLANNING GUIDANCE

SAMPLE 2 - Statewide Community Planning Group, with Regional Community Planning Groups:
LETTER OF CONCURRENCE

Date
Mr./Ms._____
Grants Management Officer
Procurement and Grants Office
Centers for Disease Control and Prevention
290 Brandywine Road
Room 300, Mailstop E-15
Atlanta, GA 30341

Dear Mr./Ms. _____:

On behalf of the statewide HIV/STD community planning group (CPG), we are confirming our concurrence with the 2004 _____ prevention plan and grant application. We believe that these documents address the prevention needs of priority populations and are being supported through the funding commitments of the health department. We feel strongly that the 2005 Plan and grant application reflect the planning efforts of the statewide HIV/STD community planning group and that a thorough review process was used to ensure concurrence. Our process included:

- The statewide resources development committee reviewed the proposed budget for 2005 at the June 2004 statewide meeting. All members of the statewide CPG received time to provide input (until early June). No one voiced opposition to the committee.
- A presentation of all regional plans to the statewide CPG ensured that the statewide CPG was aware of regional priorities. A review team composed of the statewide community co-chair, regional representatives, at-large members, and gallery participants read the plan and the regional plans to ensure that the state plan was based on the regional plans.
- A second-review team composed of the statewide community co-chair, a new set of regional representatives, at-large members, and gallery participants, read the application and reviewed regional plans to ensure that the application met CDC guidelines.
- At the September meeting of the Statewide CPG, the Resource Development Committee presented the budget, reporting that the budget adequately reflected the priorities presented in the comprehensive plan. The plan review team followed the same process. The statewide CPG voted to accept the plan. The grant application review team followed the same process, and the CPG voted to accept the application

We look forward to implementing the plan to reduce the spread of HIV in _____.

Sincerely,

State Health Department Co-Chair State Community Co-Chair
Region X Co-Chairs, Region X Co-Chairs
Region X Co-Chairs, Region X Co-Chairs

2004–2008 HIV PREVENTION COMMUNITY PLANNING GUIDANCE

SAMPLE 3 - Statewide Community Planning Group:
LETTER OF CONCURRENCE WITH RESERVATIONS

Date
Grant Management Officer
Grants Management Branch
Procurement and Grants Office
Centers for Disease Control and Prevention
290 Brandywine Road
Room 300, Mailstop E-15
Atlanta, GA 30341
Re: LETTER OF CONCURRENCE WITH RESERVATIONS

Dear Mr./Ms._____:

We concur with our health department's application with one major exception. We are concurring with concerns to the health department's application for funding. As a CPG, we feel that the health department has consistently failed to implement effective programs for Men who Have Sex with Men (MSM). We recognize that this is a difficult population to reach, however, this is the jurisdictions's number one target population (as documented in both the epidemiologic profile and our priority setting process). The CPG has stated both the need and the types of interventions that are most needed (see the Comprehensive HIV Prevention Plan, Target Populations: MSM).

Despite our reservations about the application, we feel proud of how the _____ community planning group came together with the health department and accomplished so much with such a diverse group of individuals. The_____ community planning process is truly community driven. This was reflected in the review of the health department's application. The health department distributed copies of the application to all members and each member had ten days to review the application and to respond with comments. The community co-chairs collated comments and then participated in a conference call to make the decision to concur with concerns with the health department application.

We remain united in the struggle for healthy communities!

The _____ Community Planning Group

SAMPLE 4 - Statewide Community Planning Group:
LETTER OF NONCONCURRENCE

Date
Grants Management Officer
Procurement and Grants Office
Centers for Disease Control and Prevention
290 Brandywine Road
Room 300, Mailstop E-15
Atlanta, GA 30341
Re: LETTER OF NONCONCURRENCE

Dear Mr./Ms._____:

After careful consideration of the health department's application, we have decided not to concur with that application. The application does not reflect our priorities for target populations or interventions directed to those populations. Instead, the health department application proposes funding for programs directed at the general public and a broadly targeted HIV counseling and testing program.
We do not make this decision lightly.

Our group spent many hours reviewing epidemiologic data and the results of our needs assessment to form our population priorities. We also consulted with behavioral scientists and conducted an extensive literature review to support our intervention priorities. The health department application appears not to have recognized our efforts or recommendations.

We also want to register our dismay at the health department's lack of cooperation with the review process. Initially the CPG was informed that we would have 24 hours to review the application and that budget tables would not be included in the draft copy sent for review. We were able to negotiate three days for the review, still an inadequate amount of time.

We would greatly appreciate your help in resolving this matter.

Sincerely,

Community Co-chair

2004–2008 HIV PREVENTION COMMUNITY PLANNING GUIDANCE

D

APPENDIX

HIV Prevention Community Planning: An Orientation Guide

E

Critical Attributes of HIV Prevention Community Planning

Critical HIV Prevention Community Planning Attributes

The purpose of this section is to make explicit the critical attributes of the community planning objectives. These attributes were developed through a collaborative process that has included input from a variety of prevention partners including community and health department co-chairs, community planning technical assistance providers, the National Alliance of State and Territorial AIDS Directors, and CDC staff.

This Appendix groups attributes according to the objectives of community planning. If the designated attributes of an objective for a given jurisdiction are present in a community planning process, then one may with some level of confidence say that this objective is being met.

For evaluation purposes, designated indicators (Section VI: Accountability) have been explicitly developed based on these attributes. It is important to note that jurisdictions are not required to individually report on each attribute listed here. However, in the case of a letter of nonconcurrence, programmatic reviews conducted by CDC or a jurisdiction identified as having significant community planning challenges, the jurisdiction may be asked to provide evidence of applicable attributes.

OBJECTIVE A: Implement an open recruitment process (outreach, nominations, and selection) for CPG membership. The presence of the following attributes are critical to achieving this Objective:

☐ **Attribute 1** *(Nominations)*: Presence of written procedures for nominations to the CPG.

☐ **Attribute 2** *(Nominations)*: Evidence that written procedures (above) were used for nominations to the CPG.

☐ **Attribute 3** *(Nominations)*: Evidence that a nominations committee has been established.

☐ **Attribute 4** *(Nominations)*: Evidence that nominations targeted membership gaps as identified by the community planning group.

☐ **Attribute 5** *(Selection)*: Evidence that membership decisions involve more than the health department staff.

☐ **Attribute 6** *(Selection)*: Written documentation of the process for selection of CPG members.

☐ **Attribute 7** *(Selection)*: Evidence that the process (above) was used in selection of CPG members.

OBJECTIVE B: Ensure that the CPG(s) membership is representative of the diversity of populations most at risk for HIV infection and community characteristics in the jurisdiction, and includes key professional expertise and representation from key governmental and non-governmental agencies. The presence of the following attributes are critical to achieving this Objective:

☐ **Attribute 8** *(Representation):* CPG includes: (a) members who represent populations most at risk for HIV infection as reflected in the current and projected epidemic, as documented in the prior year's epidemiologic profile, and (b) persons living with HIV/AIDS.

☐ **Attribute 9** *(Representation):* CPG membership includes members who represent the affected community in terms of race/ethnicity, gender/gender identity, sexual orientation, and geographic distribution.

☐ **Attribute 10** *(Representation):* CPG membership includes, or has access to, professional expertise in behavioral/social science, epidemiology, evaluation, and service provision.

☐ **Attribute 11** *(Representation):* CPG membership includes, or has access to, key government agencies, including: health department HIV/AIDS program and the state/local health department STD program staff.

☐ **Attribute 12** *(Representation):* CPG membership includes, or has access to, key governmental and non-governmental agencies with expertise in factors and issues relative to HIV prevention.

OBJECTIVE C: Foster a community planning process that encourages inclusion and parity among community planning members. The presence of the following attributes are critical to achieving this Objective:

☐ **Attribute 13** *(Inclusion):* Evidence of that to gain input from representatives of marginalized groups, who would be hard to recruit and/or retain as CPG members, the CPG convened ad hoc committees, panels, and/or focus groups.

☐ **Attribute 14** *(Inclusion):* Evidence that efforts were undertaken to accommodate or facilitate members who face challenging barriers (e.g., health care or economic needs) to their continued participation in the CPG.

☐ **Attribute 15** *(Inclusion):* Evidence of a clear decision-making process, including conflict of interest rules.

☐ **Attribute 16** *(Inclusion):* Evidence of an orientation, mentoring or training process for new CPG members.

☐ **Attribute 17** *(Inclusion):* Evidence that CPG meetings are open to the public and allow time for public comment.

☐ **Attribute 18** *(Parity):* Evidence of ongoing training process for all CPG members.

OBJECTIVE D: Carry out a logical, evidence-based process to determine the highest priority, population-specific prevention needs in the jurisdiction. The presence of the following attributes are critical to achieving this Objective:

☐ **Attribute 19** *(Epidemiologic Profile)*: The epidemiologic profile provides information about defined populations at high risk for HIV infection for the CPG to consider in the prioritization process.

☐ **Attribute 20** *(Epidemiologic Profile)*: Strengths and limitations of data sources used in the epidemiologic profile are described (general issues and jurisdiction-specific issues).

☐ **Attribute 21** *(Epidemiologic Profile)*: Data gaps are explicitly identified in the epidemiologic profile.

☐ **Attribute 22** *(Epidemiologic Profile)*: The epidemiologic profile contains a narrative interpretation of data presented.

☐ **Attribute 23** *(Epidemiologic Profile)*: Evidence that the epidemiologic profile was presented to the CPG members prior to the prioritization process.

☐ **Attribute 24** *(Community Services Assessment)*: The Community Services Assessment (CSA) focuses on one or more high priority populations (i.e., substantially contributing to new HIV infections in a jurisdiction) identified in the epidemiologic profile.

☐ **Attribute 25** *(Community Services Assessment)*: Data are gathered that define populations' needs in terms of knowledge, skills, attitudes, and norms.

☐ **Attribute 26** *(Community Services Assessment)*: Data are gathered that define populations' needs in terms of access to services.

☐ **Attribute 27** *(Community Services Assessment)*: The CSA details the target populations being served.

☐ **Attribute 28** *(Community Services Assessment)*: The CSA details the interventions provided to each target population.

☐ **Attribute 29** *(Community Services Assessment)*: The CSA describes the geographic coverage of interventions or programs.

☐ **Attribute 30** *(Community Services Assessment)*: The CSA was utilized in demonstrating linkages between the application and funded interventions.

☐ **Attribute 31** *(Community Services Assessment)*: Evidence that prior to the prioritization process, the CPG was provided with a summary of the CSA.

☐ **Attribute 32** *(Gap Analysis)*: The gap analysis includes data from the epidemiologic profile and CSA.

☐ **Attribute 33** *(Gap Analysis)*: A gap analysis specifically identifies both met and unmet needs.

☐ **Attribute 34** *(Gap Analysis)*: The gap analysis identifies the portion of needs being met with CDC funds.

☐ **Attribute 35** *(Gap Analysis)*: Evidence that prior to the prioritization process, the CPG was provided with a summary of the gap analysis findings.

☐ **Attribute 36** *(Gap Analysis)*: The gap analysis was utilized by the CPG in demonstrating linkages between the application and funded interventions

OBJECTIVE E: Ensure that priority target populations are based on an epidemiologic profile and a community services assessment. The presence of the following attributes are critical to achieving this Objective:

☐ **Attribute 37** *(Target Populations)*: Evidence that the size of at-risk populations was considered in setting priorities for target populations.

☐ **Attribute 38** *(Target Populations)*: Evidence that a measurement of the percentage of HIV morbidity (i.e., HIV/AIDS incidence or prevalence), if available, was considered in setting priorities for target populations.

☐ **Attribute 39** *(Target Populations)*: Evidence that the prevalence of risky behaviors in the population was considered in setting priorities for target populations.

☐ **Attribute 40** *(Target Populations)*: Target populations are defined by transmission risk, gender, age, race/ethnicity, HIV status, and geographic location.

☐ **Attribute 41** *(Target Populations)*: Target populations are rank ordered by priority, in terms of their contribution to new HIV infections.

OBJECTIVE F: Ensure that prevention activities/interventions for identified priority target populations are based on behavioral and social science, outcome effectiveness, and/or have been adequately tested with intended consumers for cultural appropriateness, relevance, and acceptability. The presence of the following attributes are critical to achieving this Objective:

☐ **Attribute 42** *(Prevention Activities/Interventions)*: Demonstrated application of existing behavioral and social science, and pre- and post-test outcome evidence (including evaluation date, when available) to show effectiveness in averting or reducing high-risk behavior within the target population.

☐ **Attribute 43** *(Prevention Activities/Interventions)*: Evidence that the prevention activity/intervention is acceptable to the target population (e.g., testing, focus groups, etc.).

☐ **Attribute 44** *(Prevention Activities/Interventions)*: Evidence that the prevention activity/intervention is feasible to implement for the intended population in the intended setting.

☐ **Attribute 45** *(Prevention Activities/Interventions)*: Evidence that the prevention activity/intervention was developed by or with input from the target population.

☐ **Attribute 46** *(Prevention Activities/Interventions)*: Prevention activities/interventions are characterized by focus, level, factors expected to affect risk, setting, and frequency/duration.

☐ **Attribute 47** *(Prevention Activities/Interventions)*: Each prevention activity/intervention is also characterized by scale and significance.

☐ **Attribute 48** *(Prevention Activities/Interventions)*: Prevention activities/interventions are prioritized by risk population and their ability to have the greatest impact on decreasing new infections.

Objective G: Demonstrate a direct relationship between the Comprehensive HIV Prevention Plan and the Health Department Application for federal HIV prevention funding. The presence of the following attributes are critical to achieving this Objective:

☐ **Attribute 49** *(Comprehensive Plan):* Explicit demonstration of linkages between the comprehensive HIV prevention plan and the health department application to CDC for federal funding.

☐ **Attribute 50** *(Comprehensive Plan):* Letter of Concurrence.

Objective H: Demonstrate a direct relationship between the Comprehensive HIV Prevention Plan and funded interventions. The presence of the following attributes are critical to achieving this Objective:

☐ **Attribute 51** *(Comprehensive Plan):* Explicit demonstration of linkages between the comprehensive HIV prevention plan and funded interventions.

☐ **Attribute 52** *(Community Services Assessment):* Explicit demonstration that the CPG has used the CSA to determine whether interventions were funded according to the comprehensive HIV prevention plan.

F

Community Planning Monitoring and Evaluation Forms

Includes:

HIV Prevention Community Planning Membership Survey

Community Planning Linkage Table Worksheet

INSTRUCTIONS FOR COMPLETING
THE COMMUNITY PLANNING MEMBERSHIP SURVEY

Purpose

The community planning membership survey is designed to gain input from community planning groups (CPGs) on their perspectives regarding the implementation and quality of the community planning process within their jurisdictions. Its purpose is to provide CDC with a picture of what is occurring in HIV Prevention Community Planning across the country and to serve as a useful tool for CPGs in improving community planning processes at the local level. The opinions of CPG members are very important for both purposes. Input from you and other CPG members will be used to guide improvements to the community planning process nationwide as well as to identify unique strengths and potential training needs within your own CPG.

Before you begin, here are a few things you should know:

■ Completion of the survey should take approximately 30-40 minutes.

■ If you are a member of more than one CPG, please fill out a survey for each CPG.

■ A "comments" section follows each group of items in the survey for you to provide additional thoughts regarding your responses or questions about particular sections of the survey.

■ Your participation in this survey is *voluntary*, and you may choose not to answer any one or more questions.

■ The information you provide will be kept *confidential*. Survey responses will be presented in an aggregate format and your individual information will not be linked to your responses.

■ If during the survey you have particular questions or come across items that are unclear, it's okay to ask for clarification from your CPG Co-chairs or other individuals who are administering the surveys. However, please also note your questions in the comments section. Your feedback is valuable and will help us make these items clearer in the future.

■ When you are finished, please return the survey to the designated individual within your CPG (i.e., CPG Co-Chair, Community Planning Coordinator, Evaluator).

■ We *greatly* appreciate your time! Your participation in this survey will help to improve the quality of the community planning process and will ultimately contribute to the development of a system to assess HIV prevention community planning nationwide.

Please note that the Office of Management and Budget (OMB) requires CDC to follow certain standards when collecting data on race and ethnicity. The standards have five categories for data on race: American Indian or Alaska Native, Asian, Black or African American, Native Hawaiian or Other Pacific Islander, and White. There are two categories for data on ethnicity: "Hispanic or Latino," and "Not Hispanic or Latino." The standards have been developed to provide a common language for uniformity and comparability in the collection and use of data on race and ethnicity by Federal agencies. (Statistical Policy Directive No. 15, Race and Ethnic Standards for Federal Statistics and Administrative Reporting, 1997) For more information, see also OMB guidance entitled Implementation of the 1997 Standards for Federal Data on Race and Ethnicity (2000) or visit the OMB website at http://www.whitehouse.gov/omb/fedreg/ombdir15.html

Thank You for Participating!

Date: _____

COMMUNITY PLANNING MEMBERSHIP SURVEY – PART I

INTRODUCTION:
The first series of items will ask about various characteristics of your CPG and some demographic information about you and the role you play as a CPG member.

Please respond to these items as openly as possible, for the most recent year during which you participated in HIV prevention community planning (i.e., July 1, 2003 through June 30, 2004). The information you provide will be kept confidential and responses to any one or more items is voluntary.

Name and type of the HIV Prevention CPG you will be referring to throughout this survey

1. Name of the HIV Prevention CPG: _____

2. Type of HIV Prevention CPG:
   ☐ Statewide planning group   ☐ Directly-funded city planning group
   ☐ Regional planning group   ☐ Other (_____)
   ☐ Local planning group

Demographic Information of CPG member

3. Age (choose one):

☐ ≤13	☐ 13-18	☐ 19-24	☐ 25-34	☐ 35-44	☐ 45+

4. Gender (choose one):

☐ Male   ☐ Female   ☐ Transgender

5. Sexual orientation

☐ Heterosexual   ☐ Gay   ☐ Lesbian   ☐ Bisexual
☐ Unknown   ☐ Other (specify): _____   ☐ No Response

6. Ethnicity (choose one): *Please note*: All members should choose an option for ethnicity. This item applies to all members regardless of your response to #7 (below).

☐ Hispanic/Latino   ☐ Non-Hispanic/Non-Latino

7. Race (Choose more than one if applicable):

☐ American Indian or Alaska Native   ☐ Native Hawaiian or Other Pacific Islander
☐ Asian   ☐ White
☐ Black or African-American   ☐ No Response

Demographic Information (cont.)

8. Type of geographic location in which you live (choose one):

- ☐ Rural: An area with a population of less that 2,500 (typically a small town or a community with a population that is widely dispersed or spread out)
- ☐ Urban non-metropolitan: An area with a population of between 2,500 and 100,000 (small to mid-size city)
- ☐ Suburb: A residential area around or outlying a city
- ☐ Urban metropolitan: An area with a population of greater than 100,000 (large city, densely populated such as New York, Los Angeles, Houston)
- ☐ Other (please specify: _____)

9. Primary areas of expertise (Select up to two, placing a ì1î next to your primary expertise area and ì2î next to your secondary area):

___ Community Representative	___ Behavioral or Social Scientist
___ Community Organization	___ Evaluation
___ PLWHA (person living with or affected by HIV/AIDS)	___ Health Planner
___ Intervention Specialist/Service Provider	___ Epidemiologist
___ Other (please specify: _____)	

10. HIV risk populations whose perspectives you represent through personal life experiences, work responsibilities, or other affiliations. (Select up to two, placing a ì1î next to your primary and ì2î next to your secondary perspective):

- ☐ Men who have sex with men and are at risk through unsafe sex
- ☐ Men who are at risk from both unsafe sex with other men and unsafe drug injection practices
- ☐ Men and women who are at risk through unsafe injection drug practices
- ☐ Men and women who are at risk through unsafe heterosexual sex with an infected partner
- ☐ Men and women who are at risk through unsafe sex with a transgender
- ☐ Men and women who are at risk from both unsafe sex with a transgender and unsafe injection drug practices
- ☐ Men and women not part of a specific population at risk for HIV

HIV/AIDS Status

11. What is your HIV serostatus?

☐ Living with HIV/AIDS   ☐ Not living with HIV/AIDS   ☐ Unknown   ☐ No Response

12. Do you have a relative, partner, or close friend who is living with HIV/AIDS or who has died from HIV/AIDS?

☐ Yes   ☐ No   ☐ Donít know

Agency Representation

13. Type of organization you represent or are affiliated with (Select up to two, placing a ì1î next to your primary affiliation and ì2î next to your secondary affiliation). If you do not represent an agency, please check ìNon-Agency/Community Representative.î

___ Faith Community	___ Health Department: HIV/AIDS	___ Mental Health
___ Minority CBO*	___ Health Department: STD	___ Homeless Services
___ Non-minority CBO	___ Substance Abuse	___ Academic Institution
___ Other Nonprofit	___ HIV Care and Social Services	___ Research Center
___ Business and Labor	___ State/Local Education Agencies	___ Corrections
___ Other (please specify): _____		___ Non-Agency/Community Rep.

*Minority CBO ñ Provides HIV Prevention services to members of racial/ethnic minority communities who are at risk for HIV infection (≥ 85% of persons served in each of the last three years were of racial/ethnic minority populations).

Agency Representation (cont.)

14. Does your primary organization receive HIV prevention funding from the state/city/territory health department?

☐ Yes ☐ No ☐ Not applicable

15. Does your secondary organization receive HIV prevention funding from the state/city/territory health department?

☐ Yes ☐ No ☐ Not applicable

General Information about the CPG

Please respond to this next set of items for the most recent year during which you participated in HIV prevention community planning (i.e., July 1, 2003 through June 30, 2004).

16. During the past planning year, how many CPG meetings (of the general membership) did you attend?	_____ # of meeting(s)
17. In what year did you become a member of the CPG you currently belong to?	_____ (i.e., 1999, 2001)

Comments/Questions

_____
_____
_____
_____
_____
_____
_____
_____

End of Part I

COMMUNITY PLANNING MEMBERSHIP SURVEY – PART II

INTRODUCTION

This next series of items asks your opinion regarding whether the objectives of community planning were met in your CPG during the most recent year of planning. Each objective is followed by a series of items that ask you to indicate your agreement or disagreement with the presence of a specific attribute or key step in the community planning process. If you are unsure about a particular item, please indicate "Don't Know."

> **INSTRUCTIONS FOR OBJECTIVE A:**
>
> This first set of items is related to Goal 1, Objective A. These items relate to how the CPG recruits and selects new members. This would include the procedures that the CPG follows to nominate and elect new members.
>
> Please complete the items under Objective A.

Goal 1: Community Planning supports broad-based community participation in HIV Prevention Planning

Objective A: Implement an open recruitment process (outreach, nominations, and selection) for CPG membership.

Please rate your agreement with each of the following statements.	Agree	Disagree	Don't Know
A1. The CPG **has** written procedures for nominations to the CPG.	☐	☐	☐
A2. The CPG **uses** the written procedures (above) for nominations to the CPG.	☐	☐	☐
A3. The CPG has established a nominations/membership committee.	☐	☐	☐
A4. CPG nominations target membership gaps identified by the members of the CPG.	☐	☐	☐
A5. Both CPG members and health department staff participate in membership decisions.	☐	☐	☐
A6. The CPG **has** written procedures for how to select CPG members.	☐	☐	☐
A7. The CPG **uses** the written procedures (above) in selection of CPG members.	☐	☐	☐
Comments/Questions			

_____

_____

_____

_____

_____

_____

_____

INSTRUCTIONS FOR OBJECTIVE B:

The goal of this next set of items is to gain information from CPG members about parity, inclusion and representation. These items will focus on the diversity of the CPG membership and whether this diversity represents the populations most at risk for HIV infection in your community.

These items will also focus on the various relationships or connections the CPG has with other key players, including other government and non-government agencies and individuals with expertise relative to HIV prevention.

Please complete the next section.

Objective B: Ensure that CPG membership is representative of the diversity of populations most at risk for HIV infection and community characteristics in the jurisdiction and includes key professional expertise and representation from key governmental and non-governmental agencies.

Please rate your agreement with each of the following statements.	Agree	Disagree	Don't Know
B1. The CPG includes members who represent each population of the current and projected epidemic as documented in the epidemiologic profile.	☐	☐	☐
B2. The CPG has expert perspective available from behavioral/social science on issues related to the community planning process.	☐	☐	☐
B3. The CPG has expert perspective available in epidemiology on issues related to the community planning process.	☐	☐	☐
B4. The CPG has expert perspective available in evaluation on issues related to the community planning process.	☐	☐	☐
B5. The CPG has expert perspective available in service provision (i.e., intervention specialists, medical providers, counselors) on issues related to the community planning process.	☐	☐	☐
B6. The CPG has expert perspective available from health department HIV/AIDS Program staff on issues related to the community planning process.	☐	☐	☐
B7. The CPG has expert perspective available from state/local health department STD program staff on issued related to the community planning process.	☐	☐	☐
B8. The CPG has expert perspective available from state/local substance abuse treatment facilities on issues related to the community planning process.	☐	☐	☐
B9. The CPG has expert perspective available from state/local HIV Care and Social Services (i.e., Ryan White Care clinics), on issues related to the community planning process.	☐	☐	☐
B10. The CPG has expert perspective available from correctional facilities, on issues related the community planning process.	☐	☐	☐
Comments/Questions			

INSTRUCTIONS FOR OBJECTIVE C:

The next section will focus on the efforts the CPG takes to ensure that all members have an opportunity to participate in the community planning process. This includes any special efforts or strategy the CPG uses to gain input from individuals, especially those whose circumstances may restrict participation (i.e., lack of transportation, health care issues). These efforts would also include the various types of training and support provided to ensure that members have the knowledge and resources needed to make informed decisions.

Please complete the next section.

Objective C: Foster a community planning process that encourages inclusion and parity among community planning members.

Please rate your agreement with each of the following statements.	Agree	Disagree	Don't Know
C1. The CPG uses various methods (i.e., focus groups, panels, or committees) to gain input from high-risk groups or individuals who would be hard to recruit and/or retain as CPG members.	☐	☐	☐
C2. The CPG undertakes efforts to assist members in their continued participation in the CPG, particularly those who face challenging barriers.	☐	☐	☐
C3. The CPG has formal procedures for making decisions and resolving disagreements among members.	☐	☐	☐
C4. Throughout the planning year, the CPG provides a process for training (i.e., presentations, speakers, capacity building workshops) for all CPG members.	☐	☐	☐
C5. The CPG provides orientation and/or other appropriate support to new CPG members.	☐	☐	☐
C6. CPG meetings are open to the public and allow time for public comment.	☐	☐	☐
Comments/Questions			

INSTRUCTIONS FOR OBJECTIVES D:

This next set of items addresses Objective D and is related to Goal 2. These items consider the resources and issues used by the CPG in defining and prioritizing risk populations and HIV prevention interventions. These resources would include the following:

1) *Epidemiologic profile:* a description of the HIV epidemic and how it impacts certain populations or geographic areas
2) *Community Services Assessment:*
    a. *needs assessment:* a process for determining the service needs of those highly impacted
    b. *resource inventory:* a detailed list of existing HIV resources and services
    c. *gap analysis:* the needs assessment and the resource inventory would be compared to each other to determine if there were populations or service needs that were not being addressed

*Both resources are used by the CPG in the priority setting process and submitted with the Comprehensive HIV Prevention Plan.

Please complete the next set of items.

F

APPENDIX

Goal 2: Community planning identifies priority HIV prevention needs in each jurisdiction.

Objective D: Carry out logical, evidence-based process to determine the highest priority, population-specific prevention needs in the jurisdiction.

Please rate your agreement with each of the following statements.	Agree	Disagree	Don't Know
D1. The epidemiologic profile (referred to here as the "epi-profile") used in the prioritization process contains the most updated* information as provided by the health department. See suggestions for updating the profile in "Integrated Guidelines for Developing Epidemiologic Profiles." HIV Prevention and Ryan White Care Act Community Planning. *DRAFT*	☐	☐	☐
D2. The epi-profile provides information about defined populations most at risk for HIV infection for the CPG to consider in the prioritization process.	☐	☐	☐
D3. Strengths and limitations of data sources used in the epi-profile are described.	☐	☐	☐
D4. The epi-profile contains a written explanation of the data presented.	☐	☐	☐
D5. The epi-profile was presented to the CPG members prior to voting on priorities.	☐	☐	☐
Comments/Questions			

_____

_____

_____

_____

_____

_____

_____

Please rate your agreement with each of the following statements.	Agree	Disagree	Don't Know
D6. The community services assessment (**referred to here as the CSA**) focuses on one or more most at risk populations identified in the epi-profile.	☐	☐	☐
D7. The CSA contains data that define populations' needs in terms of knowledge, skills, attitudes, and norms.	☐	☐	☐
D8. The CSA contains data that define populations' needs in terms of access to services.	☐	☐	☐
D9. The CSA describes the target populations being served (i.e., age, gender, race).	☐	☐	☐
D10. The CSA describes the interventions provided to each target population (i.e., types of activities, number of sessions).	☐	☐	☐
D11. The CSA describes the geographic coverage of interventions or programs.	☐	☐	☐
D12. The CSA specifically identifies both met and unmet needs.	☐	☐	☐
D13. The CSA identifies the portion of needs being met with CDC funds.	☐	☐	☐
D14. The CSA was presented to the CPG members prior to voting on priorities	☐	☐	☐
D15. The CSA was utilized in demonstrating linkages between the plan and the application.	☐	☐	☐
Comments/Questions			

INSTRUCTIONS FOR OBJECTIVE E:

This objective focuses on the issues or factors that the CPG considers when prioritizing populations at risk for HIV infection.

Please complete the next set of items.

Objective E: Ensure that priority target populations are based on an epidemiologic profile and a community services assessment.

Please rate your agreement with each of the following statements:	Agree	Disagree	Don't Know
E1. The CPG considers available information on the size (estimated total number) of the most at risk populations.	☐	☐	☐
E2. The CPG considers the level of disease burden in the most at risk populations.	☐	☐	☐
E3. The CPG considers the prevalence (frequency of occurrence or amount) of risky behaviors in the most at risk populations.	☐	☐	☐
E4. The CPG considers the priority needs of the most at risk populations (access to services, cultural/language barriers, special health care needs).	☐	☐	☐
Comments/Questions			

F

APPENDIX

INSTRUCTIONS FOR OBJECTIVE F:

This objective focuses on the issues or factors that the CPG considers when selecting particular HIV prevention activities. In this context, prevention activities are activities that have a focus on any of the following areas: behavioral interventions, structural interventions, capacity building, and information gathering.

Please complete the next set of items.

Objective F: *Ensure that prevention activities for identified priority populations are based on behavioral and social science, outcome effectiveness and/or have been adequately tested with intended consumers for culture appropriateness, relevance, and acceptability.*

Please rate your agreement with each of the following statements:.	Agree	Disagree	Don't Know
F1. The CPG considers whether the prevention activities are culturally appropriate and acceptable for the most at risk populations (i.e., through focus groups, pilot testing, reviewing studies).	☐	☐	☐
F2. The CPG considers whether implementation of the prevention activity is possible (achievable) for its intended populations and in its setting.	☐	☐	☐
F3. The CPG considers whether the prevention activities were developed by or with input from the most at risk population (i.e., key informant interviews, focus groups, surveys).	☐	☐	☐
F4. The CPG considers the known effectiveness of prevention activities in averting or reducing HIV infection (Examples may include those listed or based upon the programs in the *Compendium of HIV Prevention Programs with Evidence of Effectiveness*).* *Exact replication of programs is not always appropriate within a given jurisdiction given regional and/or population-based circumstances. "Consideration of known effectiveness" includes reviewing the literature and applying a reasonable amount of tailoring to fit local circumstances.	☐	☐	☐

Comments/Questions

_____
_____
_____
_____
_____
_____
_____
_____
_____
_____

INSTRUCTIONS FOR OBJECTIVES G-H:

This next set of items address Objectives G-H and is related to Goal 3. These items refer to the process of comparing the relationship or connection between the comprehensive HIV prevention plan, the health department's application for HIV prevention funding and the resources allocated for HIV prevention activities.

Important Note:

The first item addresses the process used to develop or update the comprehensive HIV prevention plan for *next* year and the application that will be submitted for the same year (i.e., 2004).

The second item addresses the *prior* year's comprehensive plan. It asks you to look back in time and determine whether the interventions funded during the past year corresponded to the priorities in the prior year's comprehensive HIV prevention plan.

Please complete the next set of items.

Goal 3: Community planning ensures that HIV prevention resources target priority populations and prevention activities set forth in the comprehensive HIV prevention plan.

Objective G: Demonstrate a direct relationship between the Comprehensive HIV prevention plan and the health department application for federal HIV prevention funding.

Objective H: Demonstrate a direct relationship between the Comprehensive HIV prevention plan and funded interventions/services delivered.

Please rate your agreement with each of the following statements.	Agree	Disagree	Don't Know
G-H1. Evidence of correspondence between the comprehensive plan and the health department application to CDC for federal funding was provided to the CPG.	☐	☐	☐
G-H2. Evidence of correspondence between the comprehensive plan and funded interventions/services delivered in the *prior year* was provided to the CPG.	☐	☐	☐
Comments/Questions			

Final Questions

This final section provides an opportunity for you to give additional feedback on your participation in the community planning process and to make recommendations on how to strengthen the process in the future.

_____
_____
_____
_____
_____
_____
_____
_____
_____
_____
_____
_____
_____
_____
_____
_____
_____
_____
_____
_____
_____
_____
_____

Thank You Very Much for Taking the Time to Complete this Survey

HIV PREVENTION COMMUNITY PLANNING MEMBERSHIP SURVEY REPORT

Instructions:

■ This report, to be completed by CPG co-chairs (or appropriate designee), is designed to assist CDC and health departments in assessing the implementation of HIV prevention community planning and it will also serve as a useful tool for CPGs in improving community planning processes at the local level. Please report the aggregate data requested in the suggested format and provide any additional narrative information necessary to clarify, support, or explain the survey findings.

■ Jurisdictions with multiple official planning groups should complete a separate membership grid for each official group.

■ Community Planning Group (CPG) members are those individuals who have the right to approve the jurisdiction's comprehensive plan and vote on concurrence with the jurisdiction's application to CDC for cooperative agreement funding.

■ The total number of CPG members for each table should be the same, except in tables 5b and 9b.

■ Use the "comments" section after each table to explain how individuals who are not official voting CPG members may provide representation. For example, in Table 9. "Expertise," could indicate that an epidemiologist is not a member of the CPG, but regularly participates in CPG meetings.

Name of the CPG:

Type of CPG: ☐ Statewide ☐ Directly-funded City
              ☐ Regional   ☐ Other: _____
              ☐ Local

Number of years covered by the current HIV prevention plan: _____

During the past planning year, how many meetings (general membership) were held? : _____

How many months is one term on the CPG for members? _____ # of months

Part I - Community Planning Group Membership Profile

Table 1: Age

≤ 13	13-18	19-24	25-34	35-44	45+	Unknown	Total CPG Members
							0

Comments:

Table 2: Gender

Male	Female	Transgender	Unknown	Total CPG Members
				0

Comments:

Community Planning Membership Survey

Table 3a: Race

American Indian or Alaska Native	Asian	Black or African American	Native Hawaiian/ Other Pacific Islander	White	More Than One Race*	Unknown	Total CPG Members
							0

*Please provide the total number of those who selected more than one racial category.

Comments:

Table 3b: Ethnicity

Hispanic or Latino	Not Hispanic or Latino	Unknown	Total CPG Members
			0

Comments:

F

APPENDIX

Table 4: Geographic Distribution

Urban Metropolitan Area	Urban Non-Metropolitan Area	Suburb	Rural	Unknown	Total CPG Members
					0

Comments:

Table 5a: Primary Area of Expertise[1]

Community Organization	PLWHA	Intervention Specialist/ Service Provider	Behavioral or Social Scientist	Evaluation Researcher	Health Planner	Epidemiologist	Other*	Unknown	Total CPG Members
									0

*In comments section (below), please provide examples of "Other."

Comments:

[1] All CPG members must have a primary expertise category, however they may not have a secondary expertise category.

Table 5b: Secondary Area of Expertise

Community Organization	PLWHA	Intervention Specialist/ Service Provider	Behavioral or Social Scientist	Evaluation	Health Planner	Epidemiologist	Other*	Unknown	Total CPG Members
									0

*In comments section (below), please provide examples of "Other."

Comments:

Table 6a: Primary HIV Risk Category[2]

MSM	MSM/IDU	IDU	Heterosexual	TG	TG/IDU	Non-specific or Unknown	Total CPG Members
							0

Comments:

F

APPENDIX

Table 6b: Secondary HIV Risk Category

MSM	MSM/IDU	IDU	Heterosexual	TG	TG/IDU	Non-specific or Unknown	Total CPG Members
							0

Comments:

Table 7a: Primary HIV Risk Category by Ethnicity

Category / Ethnicity	MSM	MSM/IDU	IDU	Heterosexual	TG	TG/IDU	Non-specific or Unknown	Unknown
Hispanic or Latino								
Not Hispanic or Latino								
Unknown								
Subtotal CPG Members	0	0	0	0	0	0	0	0

Comments:

Table 7b: Primary HIV Risk Category by Race

Category / Race	MSM	MSM/IDU	IDU	Heterosexual	TG	TG/IDU	Non-specific or Unknown	Unknown
American Indian or Alaska Native								
Asian								
Black or African American								
Native Hawaiian/ Other Pacific Islander								
White								
More Than One Race*								
Unknown								
Subtotal CPG Members	0	0	0	0	0	0	0	0

*Please provide the total number of those who selected more than one racial category.

Comments: (Table 7b)

F | APPENDIX

Table 8a: CPG Members Living with HIV/AIDS

Yes	No	Unknown	Total CPG Members
			0

Comments:

Table 8b: CPG Members Not Living with HIV/AIDS but Affected by HIV/AIDS

Yes	No	Unknown	Total CPG Members
			0

Comments:

Table 9a: Primary Agency/Other Representation[3]

Faith Community	Minority Board CBO	Non-minority Board CBO	Other Nonprofit	Business/ Labor	Health Department HIV/AIDS	Health Department STD	Substance Abuse	HIV Care and Social Services	State/Local Educational Agencies	Mental Health	Homeless Services	Total CPG Members
												0

Academic Institution	Research Center	Non-Agency/ Comm. Rep.	Corrections	Other*								

*In comments section (below), please provide examples of "Other" (e.g., advocate, IDU representative).

Comments:

Table 9b: Secondary Agency/Other Representation

	Faith Community	Minority Board CBO	Non-minority Board CBO	Other Nonprofit	Business/Labor	Health Department: HIV/AIDS	Health Department: STD	Substance Abuse	HIV Care and Social Services	State/Local Educational Agencies	Mental Health	Homeless Services	Total CPG Members
	Academic Institution	Research Center	Non-Agency/ Comm. Rep.	Corrections	Other⁻								0

*In comments section (below), please provide examples of "Individual" and "Other" (e.g., advocate, IDU representative).

Comments:

Part II Community Planning Membership Survey

Instructions:

- For each Objective in the survey, compute the total number of "Agree" responses and enter that number in the Objective's Column "A" below.

- Compute the total number of "Disagree" responses and enter that number in the Objective's Column "B" below.

- Total Columns "A" and "B" and enter that number in Column "C." That number represents the total number of valid responses for the items related to the Objective.

- Divide the number in Column "A" by the number in Column "C" for each Objective. That number or decimal represents the percentage of agreement to the items for the Objective, and should be entered in Column "D" for each Objective.

- The last section of the form represents the overall agreement with ALL items on the survey. For Column "A" in this section, compute the total number of "Agree" responses for all Objectives. Enter that number in Column "A."

- Compute the total number of "Disagree" responses for ALL Objectives and enter that number in Column "B."

- Total the numbers in Columns "A" and "B," and enter that number in Column "C."

- Divide the number in Column "A" by the number in Column "C." That number or decimal represents the percentage of agreement for ALL items in the survey, and should be entered in Column "D."

- Use the "comments" section after each table to explain low scores, unexpected findings, or any other information that would give CDC a more complete and accurate picture of the CPG process. An example might be that several new CPG members may have joined the group after the CPG orientation and may, as a result, "disagree" with the statement about orientation. This is important contextual information that will guide interpretation of the data submitted in this report.

Objective A: Implement an open recruitment process (outreach, nominations and selection) for CPG membership.

Column A	Column B	Column C	Column D
Total Number of "Agree" Responses to Items in "Objective A"	Total Number of "Disagree" Responses to Items in "Objective A"	Total Number of "Agree" and "Disagree" Responses to Items in "Objective A" This number represents the Total Number of Valid Responses	Percentage Agreement for Items in "Objective A"

Comments:

Objective B: Ensure that the CPG(s) membership is representative of the diversity of populations most at risk for HIV infection and community characteristics in the jurisdiction and includes key professional expertise and representation from key governmental and non-governmental agencies.

Column A	Column B	Column C	Column D
Total Number of "Agree" Responses to Items in "Objective B"	Total Number of "Disagree" Responses to Items in "Objective B"	Total Number of "Agree" and "Disagree" Responses to Items in "Objective B" This number represents the Total Number of Valid Responses	Percentage Agreement for Items in "Objective B"

Comments:

Objective C: Foster a community planning process that encourages inclusion and parity among community planning members.

Column A	Column B	Column C	Column D
Total Number of "Agree" Responses to Items in "Objective C"	Total Number of "Disagree" Responses to Items in "Objective C"	Total Number of "Agree" and "Disagree" Responses to Items in "Objective C" This number represents the Total Number of Valid Responses	Percentage Agreement for Items in "Objective C"

Comments:

Core Objective D: Carry out logical, evidence-based process to determine the highest priority, population-specific prevention needs in the jurisdiction.

Column A	Column B	Column C	Column D
Total Number of "Agree" Responses to Items in "Objective D"	Total Number of "Disagree" Responses to Items in "Objective D"	Total Number of "Agree" and "Disagree" Responses to Items in "Objective D" This number represents the Total Number of Valid Responses	Percentage Agreement for Items in "Objective D"

Comments:

F | APPENDIX

Core Objective E: Ensure that priority target populations are based on an epidemiologic profile and a community services assessment.

Column A	Column B	Column C	Column D
Total Number of "Agree" Responses to Items in "Objective E"	Total Number of "Disagree" Responses to Items in "Objective E"	Total Number of "Agree" and "Disagree" Responses to Items in "Objective E" This number represents the Total Number of Valid Responses	Percentage Agreement for Items in "Objective E"

Comments:

Core Objective F: Ensure that prevention activities for identified priority populations are based on behavioral and social science, outcome effectiveness and/or have been adequately tested with intended consumers for culture appropriateness, relevance, and acceptability.

Column A	Column B	Column C	Column D
Total Number of "Agree" Responses to Items in "Objective F"	Total Number of "Disagree" Responses to Items in "Objective F"	Total Number of "Agree" and "Disagree" Responses to Items in "Objective F" This number represents the Total Number of Valid Responses	Percentage Agreement for Items in "Objective F"

Comments:

Objective G: Demonstrate a direct relationship between the Comprehensive HIV prevention plan and the health department application for federal HIV prevention funding.

Objective H: Demonstrate a direct relationship between the Comprehensive HIV prevention plan and funded interventions/ services delivered.

Column A	Column B	Column C	Column D
Total Number of "Agree" Responses to Items in "Objectives G & H"	Total Number of "Disagree" Responses to Items in "Objectives G & H"	Total Number of "Agree" and "Disagree" Responses to Items in "Objectives G & H" This number represents the Total Number of Valid Responses	Percentage Agreement for Items in "Objectives G & H"

Comments:

Overall Percentage of Agreement

Column A	Column B	Column C	Column D
Total Number of **ALL** "Agree" Responses	Total Number of **ALL** "Disagree" Responses	Total Number of **ALL** "Agree" and "Disagree" Responses This number represents the Total Number of Valid Responses	Percentage Agreement for **ALL** Items

Date Report was completed: _____

Community Co-chair   Health Department Co-chair

F | APPENDIX

DRAFT LINKAGES TABLE WORKSHEETS

Purpose

The Linkage Tables are designed to answer the question,

"Have the community planning priorities been addressed by the health department and other funders in the community?"

The logic underlying these worksheets are as follows.

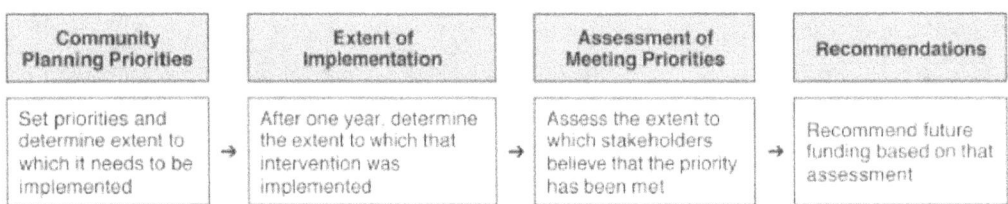

The scale of interventions is a critical aspect of the Linkage Tables. For an intervention to have an effect on the epidemic within a priority population in a jurisdiction, a certain number of people in that priority population must be served with it.

Efficacy of the Intervention (Effect Size)	x	Numbers of People Reached (Scale)	=	Effect on the Epidemic

Without a sense of the scale needed to have an effect, it is difficult to interpret the linkage between priorities and prevention activities implemented in the community. Without scale, a prevention intervention stated as "Do Group-Level Interventions for African American MSM" could be satisfied by one group being done over the course of the year for 10 men. A jurisdiction could realistically answer, "Yes, we did a Group-Level Intervention for African-American MSM." However, this may not reflect the intent or spirit of the prevention activity. The scale quantifies an estimate of how much of that intervention the community-planning group (CPG) believes is needed in their jurisdiction to do something significant about the HIV/AIDS problem there.

There are multiple types of estimates of need, but only one that is most on target for the Linkage Table worksheets. The others refer to different types of need, all of which are important for various aspects of planning, service delivery, and understanding implementation, but not as relevant as a reference point for how much service was delivered. The table below characterizes these differences.

Types of Estimates of Need		
Type of Estimate	**Example Statement about the Estimate**	**Notes**
Size of the Population With Risk Behaviors	"There are an estimated ZZZ number of people in our jurisdiction who engage in [ ] risk behavior."	This is the broadest estimate of need. It represents all those who are at risk for infection or for infecting others. This number may be much larger than the scale needed to have an effect and much larger than what can reasonably be delivered for a particular intervention.
Size of the "Reachable" Population	"Of the ZZZ people who engage in [ ] risk behavior, ZZZ - N can be reached with public health interventions."	The reachable population is a subset of the group described above. It is a loosely defined estimate of that proportion of the priority population who might feasibly be reached with one or more evaluation efforts. With respect to an estimate of scale needed, this estimate has the same limitations as noted above.
Scale/Intended Reach	"Intervention XXX should reach at least YYY people to contribute to a significant impact on the epidemic."	This is the measure of how many people need to be reached *with this particular intervention* to have a significant impact on the local epidemic. It may be a subset of the reachable population.
Intervention Plan Estimates	"With CDC funds, we intend to fund grantees that will serve at least YYY people with intervention XXX."	This estimate is the one provided by Health Departments that portrays the number of clients they expect to reach with particular intervention type through providers and staff *receiving Health Department funds*. This estimate may be a subset of the scale estimate considered broadly for the jurisdiction, as it is based on funding plans and availability of funds (whereas scale is a measure of what is needed, overall, to show an effect).

- Linkage Tables do NOT address whether the health department has funded prevention activities that were not selected as priorities by the CPG. Thus, in terms of the concurrence process, the linkage tables address one critical part (i.e. the extent to which priorities have been addressed), but not the overall relationship of the health department's proposed funding to the priorities and non-priorities.

Completing Linkage Table Worksheet #1

The purpose of Linkage Table #1 is to assess the correspondence between the target populations and interventions proposed in the HIV Prevention Plan that was developed (or updated) in the prior year and the actual services delivered to this population. The reference points for this worksheet are the priority populations and interventions derived for each jurisdiction. In particular, information from the *Priority Population Summary Worksheet* and the *Prevention Intervention/Other Supporting Activity Summary Worksheet* can be used to complete items (1)–(7) of this worksheet. The remaining items, (8a) –(8d) require judgments to be made by Health Department staff[1].

---

[1] Completion of this report is a Health Department responsibility; Health Departments may include other partners in this process at their discretion. CPGs may find a similar process instructive for helping assess whether priorities have been addressed throughout the community.

1. **Name of priority population.** This is the same name that was provided in the *Priority Population Summary Worksheet*, Field #1 "Priority Population."

2. **Estimated size of population #1.** In item **(2a)**, provide an estimate of the number of persons in the target population that are at risk for infection or for infecting others. This number should relate to the population overall and not to the amount of this intervention needed for the population. For item **(2b)**, indicate if this number refers to the "Total Size of the Population at Risk" or "Size of the Reachable Population".

3. **Name of intervention #1 for this population.** This is the same name that was provided in the *Prevention Intervention/Other Supporting Activity Summary Worksheet*, "Name of Prevention Intervention/Other Supporting Activity."

4. **Scale and Significance.** The number of members of the priority population who needed to be reached by this prevention intervention in order to make a measurable contribution to influencing the epidemic. This number corresponds to the item, "Scale and Significance," on the *Prevention Intervention/Other Supporting Activity Summary Worksheet*. The table above shows other types of estimates that might be made and the potential limitations of each.

5. **Number of clients reached by Health Department staff and their grantees receiving CDC funds.** If grantee received any amount of CDC funds, include all clients reached by that grantee's intervention, regardless of funding sources.

6. **Number of clients reached by agencies that receive no CDC funding through the health department.** This column includes estimates of the numbers of clients reached by interventions run by agencies meeting at least one of the following criteria:

   ☐ Health Department funding without CDC funds (work performed by HD staff or their grantees)
   ☐ CDC directly-funded CBO which are not also funded by HD
   ☐ Interventions receiving neither Health Department nor CDC funding

7. **Total Estimated Numbers of Clients Reached.** This column is simply the total of columns (5) and (6). It represents the total estimated number of clients served in the jurisdiction with a certain type of intervention for a given priority population by all providers in the jurisdiction.

8. **Health Department's Assessment of the Extent to Which Community Planning Priorities Have Been Addressed.** This step entails the comparison of the scale of the intended intervention (4) to the total number of clients reached by that type of intervention in the prior year (7).

   All respondents should answer (8a). If the response to (8a) is "No" (i.e. the intervention reach was not adequate for the population with respect to the intended scale), then items (8b), (8c), and (8d) should be answered.

Completing Linkage Table Worksheet #2

The purpose of Linkage Table #2 is to assess the correspondence between the target populations and interventions that are prioritized in the newly developed or updated HIV Prevention Plan and the Health Department's HIV Prevention application for funding. The reference points for this worksheet are the new priority populations and interventions as prioritized by the CPG and completed for each jurisdiction. In particular, information from the *Priority Population Summary Worksheet* and the *Prevention Intervention/Other Supporting Activity Summary Worksheet* can be used to complete items (1)-(4) of this worksheet.

1. **Name of priority population.** This is the same name that is proposed in the *Priority Population Summary Worksheet*, "Priority Population."

2. **Estimated size of population #1.** In item **(2a)**, provide an estimate of the number of persons in the target population that are at risk for infection or for infecting others. This number should relate to the population overall and not to the amount of this intervention needed for the population. For item **(2b)** indicate if this number refers to the "Total Size of the Population at Risk" or "Size of the Reachable Population".

3. **Name of intervention #1 for this population.** This is the same name that is proposed in the *Prevention Intervention/Other Supporting Activity Summary Worksheet*, "Name of Prevention Intervention/Other Supporting Activity".

4. **Scale and Significance.** The number of members of the priority population who would need to be reached by this prevention intervention in order to make a measurable contribution to influencing the epidemic. This number corresponds to the item, "Scale and Significance," on the *Prevention Intervention/Other Supporting Activity Summary Worksheet*.

5. **Consideration of Additional Factors.** This step entails a review of current data collection and issues surrounding these data including whether changes were made to the priority populations and interventions in the prior Comprehensive Plan, an assessment of data collected in the previous year and completed for Linkage Table #1, partial year data collected as of January 1st of the current year, federal or state budget constraints, and other contextual factors that may impact the way interventions are being delivered to this population.

6. Health Department Recommendations for Use of CDC Funds.

Based on the responses to items (5a)– (5e), Health Department staff make recommendations about the disposition of future funding for this intervention. Select one recommendation from items (6a)–(6e).

DRAFT LINKAGE TABLE WORKSHEET TEMPLATE #1

Linkages between the Comprehensive HIV Prevention Plan and Actual Service Delivery

Community Plan Year: _____

Table A. Population/Intervention

Describe the scale and size of the population intended to be reached by this intervention as stated in the prior year's Comprehensive Plan

(1) Target Population: #1 (fill in name)	(2a) Estimated size of Population #1	(3) Intervention: #1 (fill in name)	(4) Scale of Intervention #1
_____	(2b) Type of Estimated size (choose one) ☐ Total or ☐ Reachable	_____	_____

Table B. Estimate of Reach

Estimated Numbers of Clients Reached During Previous Year Using This Intervention

(5) Number of clients reached by Health Department staff and their grantees receiving CDC funds	(6) Number of clients reached by agencies that receive no CDC funding through the health department	(7) Total Estimated Numbers of Clients Reached (5) + (6)
_____	_____	_____

Table C. Assessment of Linkages

Health Department's Assessment of the Extent to Which Community Planning Priorities Have Been Addressed

(8a) Intervention reach was adequate for the population	☐ Y ☐ N
If "No" to 7a, then answer each of the following questions:	
(8b) Intervention existed, but more clients needed to be reached by the existing agencies	☐ Y ☐ N
(8c) Intervention existed, but more agencies needed to be funded to reach more clients	☐ Y ☐ N
(8d) If intervention was not implemented, briefly describe the reasons	_____

DRAFT LINKAGE TABLE WORKSHEET TEMPLATE #2
Linkages between the Comprehensive Plan and the HIV Prevention Application

Community Plan Year: _____

Table A. Population/Intervention
Describe the scale and size of the population intended to be reached by this intervention as stated in the current year's Comprehensive Plan

Target Population: #1 (fill in name) _____	(2a) Estimated size of Population #1	(3) Intervention: #1 (fill in name)	(4) Scale of Intervention #1: _____
	(2b) Type of Estimated size (choose one) ☐ Total or ☐ Reachable		

Table B. Consideration of Additional Factors
Health Department's Consideration of Data Collection to Date

(5a) Changes in priorities: The priorities/scale of interventions has changed	☐ Y ☐ N	
(5b) Assessment of Previous Year's Data: Data collected in the previous year (Linkage Table #1) reveals information that may impact future recommendations.	☐ Y ☐ N	
(5c) Partial year data: Data collected since January 1st of the current year reveals information that may impact future recommendations.	☐ Y ☐ N	
(5d) Budget Constraints: Federal or state budget/policy decisions impact or restrict the ability to fund interventions for the population(s).	☐ Y ☐ N	
(5e) Other Factors?: (Please specify) _____	☐ Y ☐ N	

Table C. Recommendations
Health Department Recommendations for Use of CDC Funds

CDC funds will be used to: (check one) (Based on the responses to the items in Table B, Health Department staff make recommendations about the disposition of future funding for this intervention)		
	(6a) Continue intervention at roughly current level	☐ Y ☐ N
	(6b) Intervention will be expanded	☐ Y ☐ N
	(6c) Intervention will be funded for first time	☐ Y ☐ N
	(6d) No funding is available for this intervention	☐ Y ☐ N
	(6e) Intervention cannot be funded with Federal Resources	☐ Y ☐ N

G

Additional Resources for Community Planning Groups

CDC National TA Providers' Network

The Centers for Disease Control and Prevention (CDC) has created a network of TA providers to support HIV prevention community planning across the CDC-funded project areas. Whether your CPG needs local, regional, or national level TA, the TA Providers' Network is equipped to provide you customized support.

The organizations funded by CDC to provide TA to CPGs and their contact information include:

Academy for Educational Development
1825 Connecticut Avenue, NW
Washington, DC 20009
Contact: Nickie Bazell
Tel: (202) 884-8149
E-mail: nbazell@aed.org
Websites: **www.healthstrategies.org** or **www.hivaidsta.org**

Asian and Pacific Islander American Health Forum (APIAHF)
450 Sutter, Suite 600
San Francisco, CA 94108
Contact: ManChui Leung or Ed Tepporn
Tel: (415) 568-3307 or (415) 568-3309
E-mail: mleung@apiahf.org or etepporn@apiahf.org
Website: **www.apiahf.org**

Behavioral and Social Science Volunteer (BSSV) Program

Office on AIDS, American Psychological Association

750 First Street, NE

Washington, DC 20002-4242

Contact: E. Duane Wilkerson, MPH

Tel: (202) 218-3993 or 1-877-754-1404

E-mail: dwilkerson10@comcast.net

Website: **www.apa.org/pi/aids/bssv.html**

Inter-Tribal Council of Arizona (ITCA)

2214 North Central Avenue, Suite 100

Phoenix, AZ 85004

Contact: Michelle Sabori

Tel: (602) 302-1557

E-mail: michelle.sabori@itcaonline.com

Website: **www.itcaonline.com**

National AIDS Education & Services for Minorities (NAESM)

2001 Martin Luther King, Jr. Drive, Suite 602

Atlanta, GA 30310

Contact: Donato C. Clarke

Tel: (404) 753-2900

E-mail: dclarke@naesmonline.org

Website: **www.naesmonline.org**

National Alliance of State and Territorial AIDS Directors (NASTAD)

444 North Capitol Street, NW, Suite 339

Washington, DC 20001

Contact: Connie Jorstad

Tel: (202) 434-8090

E-mail: cjorstad@nastad.org

Website: **www.nastad.org**

National Association of People with AIDS (NAPWA)

1413 K Street, NW, Suite 700

Washington, DC 20005

Contact: Keith Folger

Tel: (202) 898-0414

E-mail: kfolger@napwa.org

Website: **www.napwa.org**

US-Mexico Border Health Association (USMBHA)
5400 Suncrest Drive, Suite C-5
El Paso, TX 79912
Contact: Maria Chaparro
Tel: (915) 833-6450 x20
E-mail: chaparrm@usmbha.org
Website: **www.usmbha.org**

Your CDC Project Officer is also a key element for successful TA. CDC Project Officers can help you diagnose your TA needs, refer and link you to other resources. Accessing your CDC Project Officer is easy. If you do not have his/her direct number, or are unsure of who your Project Officer is, please call the main number: (404) 639-5230.

Important Websites

Access a variety of community planning tools, materials, peer samples and more at:
www.hivaidsta.org/

Access CDC resources via the internet at:
www.cdc.gov/hiv/dhap.htm

The *Guidance for HIV Prevention Community Planning* can be found at:
www.cdc.gov/hiv/pubs/guidelines.htm and at www.hivaidsta.org

Learn more about the Advancing HIV Prevention (AHP) Initiative at:
www.cdc.gov/hiv/partners/ahp.htm

Find out more about the diffusion of effective behavioral interventions at:
www.effectiveinterventions.org

Order a variety of materials and resources from the National Prevention Information Network (NPIN) at:
www.cdcnpin.org/

Community Planning-Related Materials

Asians & Pacific Islanders in Community Planning Groups Manual (APIAHF) [Available at **www.apiahf.org/resources/index.htm**]

Assessing the Need for HIV Prevention Services: A Guide for Community Planning Groups (AED) August 1999. [NPIN Inventory #D153 or available at **www.hivaidsta.org**]

Bright Ideas: Innovative or Promising Practices in HIV Prevention and HIV Prevention Community Planning 2000, 2001, and 2002 (NASTAD and AED) [Available at **www.nastad.org** or **www.hivaidsta.org**]

Facilitating Meetings: A Guide for Community Planning Groups (AED) July 2001. [NPIN Inventory #D162 or Available at **www.hivaidsta.org**]

Integrated Guidelines for Developing Epidemiological Profiles: HIV Prevention and Ryan White Care Act Community Planning (CDC) 2004. [Available at **www.cdc.gov/hiv/epi_guidelines.htm** or **www.hivaidsta.org**]

NASTAD Issue Brief: State HIV Prevention Evaluation Systems 2000. [Available at **www.nastad.org**]

Orientation to Community Planning for Local Health Departments (NASTAD) 1998. [Available at **www.nastad.org**]

Principles of HIV Prevention with Positives (NAPWA) 2004. [Available at **www.napwa.org**]

Self Assessment Tool for Community Planning Groups (AED) May 1995. [NPIN Inventory #D202 or available at **www.hivaidsta.org**]

Setting HIV Prevention Priorities: A Guide for Community Planning Groups (AED) October 2000 [NPIN Inventory #D340 or available at **www.hivaidsta.org**]

Si Se Puede (USMBHA) 2004 [available at: **www.usmbha.org/english/projects/enlaces/Si_Se_Puede_ENGL.pdf**]

The State of Latinos in HIV Prevention Community Planning: A Briefing and Call to Action, March 2002. [Available at **www.hivaidsta.org**]

Viral Hepatitis and HIV: A Primer for Community Planning Groups (NASTAD) October 2002. [Available at **www.nastad.org**]

Some materials may be ordered from NPIN by accessing their website at: www.cdcnpin.org or by calling 1-800-458-5231.

www.ingramcontent.com/pod-product-compliance
Lightning Source LLC
Chambersburg PA
CBHW080304180526
45167CB00006B/2665

9781499696325